Truth has to be caught, not taught.

The best preparation I've come across is an open mind from a deep desire to live fully, an innate trust in ourselves or god or the universe to see the commonly unseen, to hear the commonly unheard and know the commonly unknown that we may take action. This preparation blossoms with the camaraderie of like-minded individuals who share their best, knowing our paths are individual.

—Sharon Williams Prahl

The Iodine Crisis

What You Don't Know About Iodine Can Wreck Your Life

Lynne Farrow

THE IODINE CRISIS:
What You Don't Know About Iodine Can Wreck Your Life
By Lynne Farrow

Books may be purchased by contacting Devon Press at:

DevonPressNY@aol.com

Cover Design: Nick Zelinger (NZ Graphics)
Interior Design: Ronnie Moore (Westype Publishing Services, Inc.)
Publisher: Devon Press
Editor: John Maling (Editing By John)
Manuscript and Cover Consultant: Judith Briles (The Book Shepherd)

Library of Congress Catalog Number: 2012956255
ISBN: 978-0-9860320-0-4

1. Iodine Deficiency. 2. Breast Cancer. 3. Health. 4. Nutrition.
5. Alternative Medicine. 6. Disease.

First Edition   10   9   8   7   6
Printed in USA

For Earl Foley

Table of Contents

Acknowledgments

When investigating a complex subject, an author meets many people who offer leads and information. You never know where you will end up or who will help. You never know what burning questions the detective work will raise as the mystery deepens. More than once, I asked myself, how did I get here? Why am I reading about iodine and syphilis in the 1800s? Why did I just buy a Civil War iodine canteen from eBay? How can this information ever help people in the present day? Who cares about iodine anyway? Fortunately, the global village that is the iodine online community cares and has created a bounty of resources that keeps growing. There are many to thank.

The Iodine Project founded by the pioneering work of Guy E. Abraham, MD, David Brownstein, MD, and Jorge Flechas, MD, created the touchstone for the iodine research which followed. I and others express our profound indebtedness to these physicians for not only revolutionary thinking but for transforming so many people's lives. The legacy lives on. I hope this book will exist as just one of many which examine the Iodine Project's significance to medical history.

Lucky for me, many other non-doctors shared my enthusiasm for chasing down the questions: Where did Iodine come from? Why did it disappear? How can we revive the information of The Golden Age of Iodine? We call this obsession *The Abraham Effect* because Dr. Guy Abraham, the father of the Iodine Movement, infected us with the incurable curiosity about iodine.

I'm indebted to many who inspired and supported my effort to write *The Iodine Crisis*. The book could not exist without the curiosity and research expertise of the online iodine groups: The Curezone Iodine Forum moderated by Steve "Trapper" Wilson, Laura Olsson and Chris C. Vulcanel, and the Yahoo Iodine Group founded by Iodine pioneer Zoe Alexander. Fred Van, thank you for your help in spreading the iodine information, gathering resources and compiling iodine stories.

Patient-to-patient experts Janie Bowthorpe, Sandra Anderson and Deb Anderson Eastman have left me an exemplary body of written work which I learn from everyday.

I would like to acknowledge our team at Breast Cancer Think Tank, the online discussion group of Breast Cancer Choices which provided so much information, experimentation and kindness during the years we have been exploring iodine. Thank you, Sally Gould, for your work helping with the website and research at *www.BreastCancerChoices.org*.

A big thank you to those who read the manuscript and offered their inspired criticism and suggestions. David Brownstein, MD, Kathleen Blake, Victoria Baker, Laura Olsson, Steve "Trapper" Wilson and Robin Stamm. I hope I captured the precious offerings you gave me. If not, any mistakes that remain are mine alone.

Lynn Razaitis, my friend and long time Iodinista, thank you for your wise guidance on the book from start to finish. I look forward to working with you on *www.IodineResearch.com*. Thank you for helping make sure the legacy of iodine will never get lost again.

Earl Foley and Ginny Kubler, thank you for your wise counsel and patience. You know how much of yourselves ended up on the pages. Gerry Simons, PA, thank you for your expertise as our local Iodine Literate Practitioner. Your brilliance and kindness turned the most challenging of times into a blessing.

Thank you to organizations such as Weston A. Price Foundation, The American College for Advancement in Medicine, The Cancer Control Society and The American Academy of Anti-Aging Medicine for getting the iodine message out there early. A special acknowledgement to Ann Fonfa and the mother ship of patient-to-patient cancer information, The Annie Appleseed Project which has been committed to reporting iodine information since the beginning. Mary Mucci of *Long Island Naturally*, the New York area owes you an award for breaking the Iodine Crisis and other stories on your show. To my friends at the Amagansett Library, I am in your debt.

Lastly, but most importantly, I'm honored by the many people who offered their iodine success stories to this book. You changed my life. You will change the lives of those who read your heartfelt words. The legacy of your stories lives on.

Foreword

The Iodine Crises: What You Don't Know About Iodine Can Wreck Your Life is a much needed book. Lynne Farrow has written an easy-to-read book that will help many who suffer from common medical ailments including fatigue, brain fog, thyroid disorders and breast disease. Ms. Farrow's description of the benefits of iodine therapy makes for compelling reading. Furthermore, this book describes the long history of iodine usage in medicine and why iodine has fallen out of favor with conventional medicine.

Lynne describes her own journey from becoming ill to obtaining good health. After a myriad of complaints, she was diagnosed with breast cancer. She gives her first-hand account of her experiences with oncologists and other doctors. Lynne was not satisfied with the information her conventional doctors were providing her. They could not answer her questions about why their recommended treatment plan would be the best option for her. Being a journalist, Lynne did her own research into breast cancer and found that iodine deficiency may be a big missing link into why so many women are being diagnosed with cancer. This book describes that journey and presents the information about iodine and breast cancer that anyone can understand.

There is a plethora of research relating iodine deficiency to breast diseases including breast cancer. In fact, the research dates back well over 70 years. Yet, conventional medicine is stuck in their model of surgery, chemotherapy, hormonal therapy, and radiation, all of which have done almost nothing to change the course of the illness in over 70 years. In fact, the only thing changing over the last 70 years is that more and more women—nearly 1 in 7—are being diagnosed with breast cancer. After finding the research relating iodine deficiency to breast cancer, Lynne took matters into her own hands and started supplementing with iodine. She immediately felt better and had many positive health benefits which she describes in the book. After this experience, Lynne was off to the races and began her quest to inform people about iodine. This path led her to found Breast Cancer Choices, Inc., which I have referred many patients to.

The most striking part of this book are the numerous case studies. From fatigue to psoriasis, headaches and cancer, people have sent Lynne their personal story about how iodine therapy improved their health. Many of the stories may seem unbelievable. However, they are not to me. I have been prescribing iodine for well over 10 years. I hear similar stories from my patients on a daily basis.

Unfortunately, for mosf patients their doctor has no knowledge about iodine therapy. In fact, most doctors think iodine is a dangerous substance that should be avoided. I should know. I have been writing and lecturing to doctors for years about the benefits of iodine. I can assure you that it is difficult to get a doctor interested in iodine therapy. They don't seem to understand that iodine is an essential ingredient—that life itself is not possible without adequate iodine levels.

Over the last 40 years, iodine levels have declined over 50 percent. The consequences of this decline are severe—including epidemic increases in illnesses of the breast, thyroid, ovaries, uterus, and prostate. Unless conventional medicine devotes its vast resources to searching for underlying causes of these illnesses we will continue to see suboptimal results with their therapies.

Conventional medicine has truly failed us all in its lack of concern for what is actually causing this epidemic rise in illness. It continues to be stuck in a diagnostic and treatment mode. Ultimately, we will not make consistent and definitive progress against these illnesses unless we understand what the underlying causes behind them are. I feel the large increase in chronic illnesses could be explained by deficiencies of essential nutrients, hormonal imbalances, and an increased exposure to toxic elements.

The resources section of this book tells you how to test for iodine deficiency and how to avoid problems when taking iodine. I hear complaints from some of my colleagues that iodine causes side effects. They are right—anything, iodine therapy included, can cause adverse effects. However, the correct use of iodine is not associated with too many adverse effects. The information that Lynne has written in *The Iodine Crisis* can teach you how to minimize side effects with iodine. These are the same steps I recommend to my patients.

I believe this book should be on every bookshelf. The information found in it can help you and your family avoid a preventable health problem. I highly recommend this book to anyone interested in improving their health.

—David Brownstein, M.D.
www.DrBrownstein.com
Author of 11 books including:
Iodine: Why You Need It, Why You Can't Live Without It
Overcoming Thyroid Disorders
Salt Your Way to Health

Introduction

Everybody thinks they know what iodine is. Everybody's wrong.

—Earl Foley

Iodine deficiency wrecked my life. For years I endured headaches with brain fog so bad that I lost my driver's license for speeding through stop signs. I slept so much my family called me Rip Van Winkle, and I could no longer work full time, even with caffeine and painkillers. I went from teaching college full time to working as a journalist part time. I grew overweight from an undiagnosed thyroid disorder and finally, when I thought my life couldn't get worse, I was diagnosed with a life threatening disease.

By some turn of fate, Iodine came into my life at just the right time. Dr. Sherri Tenpenny, a doctor I ran into casually at a medical conference, mentioned iodine for fibrocystic breast disease. I was intrigued but skeptical. After all, *iodine*? Surely, she didn't mean that brown antiseptic bottle in the medicine chest? What was iodine anyway? Didn't we get enough iodine from iodized salt?

Here's where the medical detective story starts. I decided to research iodine in the most conservative way; I started with the bounty of medical studies buried in the National Library of Medicine. Then, I ratcheted up the investigation and hunted down old and out-of-print medical books. I acquired antique iodine products from eBay, some with the instructions still intact. When a pharmacist's ledger, dated 1901, went to auction, I snapped it up. Sure enough, it was filled with countless iodine prescriptions. Records of iodine medicine stretched around the globe, going back a hundred and fifty years as a "universal medicine," and further—15,000 years—in its earlier form as seaweed. Archaeology records documented how prehistoric peoples hoarded certain seaweeds. In hopes of solving the mystery, I began creating an Iodine Time-line to recreate the series of events leading up to the time iodine vanished from common use. My intention was to recreate events leading up to the disappearance of iodine.

Why didn't somebody speak up when iodine suddenly went missing from the medical arsenal? The plot thickened when I discovered iodine was called "dangerous" by a research duo in 1948. Their opinion was contradicted by all the previous years when iodine was used liberally for everything from syphilis to breast cancer. No matter. Somehow iodine's historic benefits were suddenly snatched from the medical text books and largely banned from human research. Why? Who stole iodine?

Why did iodine-fortified bread also disappear in the 1970s? Could something in our environment be working to purge iodine? Why do people excrete half as much iodine in their urine now than 40 years ago? Is there a conspiracy here or just goofy negligence? While I was sleuthing the mystery of who stole iodine, I concluded I'd researched enough to determine that iodine was safe to consume in larger doses than the government-published daily requirement.

One morning I started the day by swallowing 50 mg of Lugol's iodine tablets. Boing! My brain came to life. Brain fog vanished. In the months that followed, all the other conditions plaguing me disappeared. My energy improved and my weight normalized. I was no longer so cold I needed to wear two pair of socks. Even superficial things improved. I used to slather my dry hands with hand lotion, day and night. Now, I can't imagine why my hands ever needed extra moisture. The iodine experience seemed too good to be true. If iodine was so great, why didn't everybody know about it?

How could one cheap nutrient reverse so many conditions? How did I get so iodine deficient anyway? I had always eaten seafood and iodized salt. What happened to the iodine in my food? Where was it going?

Then I discovered the newly minted Iodine Project founded by pioneer iodine doctors, Abraham, Brownstein and Flechas. Here was the mother lode of iodine detective work! The doctors were already on the case of iodine deficiency and had been quietly and carefully piling up documentation. On the internet, the first iodine experimenters started to appear. More doctors familiarized themselves with iodine and tried it themselves. Online groups formed to discuss and investigate taking iodine.

So many people reported benefits and swapped information that we tried to publish Frequently Asked Questions to lay out the information. We created online resources to help those new to iodine.

Predictably, skepticism reared its ugly head with online hecklers predicting that, since iodine was a "poison," soon we would all die. Some reported temporary side-effects, but no one could argue with success stories and the reversal of profound medical complaints. How many others had iodine supplementation helped? When more and more websites and doctors began to report the benefits of iodine, we began to realize a grass roots movement had emerged challenging the current theory that iodine was toxic.

My detective work uncovered evidence iodine had been used in one form or another for 15,000 years. The long medical anthropology of iodine validated its effectiveness. Iodine wasn't *alternative* medicine, it was *traditional* medicine that had been lost.

The plot thickened again when I discovered the anti-iodine element, bromine, was added to flour at the same time iodine was removed—in the 1970s. Iodine disappeared just as bromines came charging in. Besides bread and flour, bromine chemicals became an environmental hazard as they were added to mattresses, foods and other consumer products, purging much of our dietary iodine.

So what do we have? *A perfect storm for an iodine deficiency crisis.* How did the perfect storm scenario manifest? For starters, thyroid and breast disease skyrocketed between 1970 and 2000. Lower iodine levels means IQ levels dropping and obesity rates rising. The iodine crisis made us sick, fat and stupid. Think this conclusion is theoretical? Ask the people besides myself who were all three—sick, fat and stupid. Many of their stories populate this book.

The stories show exactly how people have benefited from iodine, whether it's a little or a lot. History tells us when you let people speak in their own words, a revolution begins. Thus, the many first-hand iodine reports carry the message better than any second-hand description could. Read them. The personal stories will touch your heart.

In my role as director of a nonprofit that investigates iodine as a healing strategy, I get emails from all over the world with stories about iodine. Wendy Farrow (no relation) from Canada, a patient in the 1980s of the late iodine investigator, Dr. W.R. Ghent, discovered our website and we were able to put together lost stories. A Russian immigrant even contacted me about how iodine was inhaled in Russia to keep germs from respiratory tracts when travelling. People email me before-and-after photographs, thermograms and mammogram films. The success stories keep piling up.

We can't let the stories of the Iodine Movement and its founders be lost to the vapors of history. Someone had to write about how the movement started and how it changed the way we think about arbitrary medical consensus. I've done my best to piece together who did what and when. When Dr. Guy Abraham launched the Iodine Movement, he was unaware of the significance of his feat. Many of us who were the beneficiaries of his revolutionary thinking, believe the Nobel Prize is not good enough for him. But we are willing to settle.

Lastly, *The Iodine Crisis* was written because those interested in iodine need a place to find the frequently asked questions and the answers that have developed over the years. *The Iodine Crisis: What You Don't Know About Iodine Can Wreck Your Life* serves as a patient-to-patient guide—lessons learned on the barricades. The information contained in the book makes no pretense of being medical advice. Please take the reporting in the journalistic spirit with which it is intended. Spread the word. Lend this book to your doctor. Let's continue to learn from each other.

Part 1

Finding the Iodine Solution— My Journey

Chapter One

Childhood Curiosity and Discovery

Study hard what interests you the most in the most undisciplined, irreverent and original manner possible.

—Richard P. Feynman

When I was ten months old, my parents rented a bungalow at the New Jersey shore. They set me on the sand and gave me a yellow plastic shovel.

"Dig," they said.

That was all I needed to stay transfixed for over an hour, digging in the sand, looking at the waves roll in, watching the water mysteriously sink into the sand as streaks of plant life piled up and sand crabs scurried. I remained so entranced that my parents later told me they worried I might be "slow." Every year we came back for two weeks and each year I grew more curious as my little legs carried me farther. Eventually they gave me a yellow pail for collecting my finds.

In New Jersey, we don't call the seashore "the beach." It's called the "shore" as in "let's go down to the shore." This is because the shore is more than the beach of crashing waves and suntanned bathers. The shore is a terrestrial wonderland with the bays and inlets wandering into curious backwaters. Follow a stream of salt water and you find tide pools and salt marshes filled with birds and plant life so ornate, humans could not imagine them without seeing them first hand. With my magic yellow pail and shovel, the earth opened up to me.

When I grew a few years older, going for a walk at the shore meant I never knew where to direct my eyes. What was the embarrassment of gifts deposited at my feet? The bird eggs, the seaweeds in more shades of green than I had ever seen, the intricate seashells and edible mussels tangled in sea lettuce. Why did some seaweed look like red hair? I still remember what being close to the ground felt like, examining each bit of sea-driven mystery in my hand.

"You mean I can keep this shell?" I asked. "Can I take the seaweed home?" How could any object so precious and magical be free or just left out in nature for the taking? Looking ceased being enough. My father started turning over what we found along the beach. When he turned over shells, sand crabs would scurry. He would turn over rocks and find cases of eggs.

"The Indians ate these," my father said, when I dug up a clam.

"You can eat that," he said when we found bladderwrack seaweed. "Lots of vitamins."

I learned an important lesson from this second step of exploring: you didn't need to restrict yourself to looking, then moving on. You could turn over shells, look under rocks. Active participants can learn more than mere observers.

My parents encouraged my curiosity and bought me a small Golden Book titled *Seashores* which I memorized without realizing it because I couldn't stop looking at the pictures. From the title I learned that the "things" I brought home from the shore weren't just things, but a vast system of living beings. Where did all these shells and seaweeds come from? How did they fit together? The book taught me that a curiosity needn't be idle or instant, that it could take you on a long journey and open up far-ranging worlds. If it were possible to radiocarbon date the beginning of my love affair with curiosity, I would write the date my parents put *Seashores* in my hand. Little did I know that my childhood love and obsession would lead to my eventual success in pursuing the iodine mystery.

Childhood "Training" Pays Off— Curiosity Did Not Kill the Cat

Fast forward several decades.

As a grown-up, my obsession with all things marine persists, but I could never predict a childhood of sand-digging would reinvent itself decades later in a mission to learn about iodine. Learning about anything always puzzled me. I never knew the right way to learn, so I just waded in and tried to connect the dots. This served me well in my academic and journalism careers where I discovered a learnable process called "fact checking"— finding the sources of information.

Wise mentors schooled me in how to ask better questions and how to push forward further *to ask questions of questions.*

Asking, "What's the source and function of this information?" became a skill I honed, a habit, even a reflex. These skills served me well. That is, *until I lost them.*

As a young adult, I was not well, and in my thirties I began to feel worse and worse. Headaches which had been a problem since my twenties suddenly became an everyday occurrence.

I went to a series of headache clinics around the US. A series of other diagnoses came in: hypoglycemia, adrenal weakness, hypothyroidism, chronic fatigue, candida, multiple chemical sensitivities, ovarian cysts, fibrocystic breast disease. I put on extra weight. I felt cold all the time and was a challenge to live with because I was always hungry or looking for my vial of Darvocet.

The chronic, mysterious complaints became very isolating to me because all my family members and friends seemed healthy. But in the various doctor's offices I visited, I met a lot of people like me. Their individual complaints may have been arranged in a different order of priority, but there were a lot of sick people out there searching and not getting results. Some very candid doctors said they didn't know how to treat us. Although they meant well, I grew frustrated with them. On TV, every illness came with a dramatic diagnosis and instant cure. Why couldn't these doctors find the answer for me? How many patients were out there coping, day-to-day, with no hope in sight?

Meanwhile, I tried to impersonate a healthy person, both socially and in business. Here was the stop-gap solution. I only picked jobs where I could control the amount of time I spent in public. My full-time college teaching job only required three days a week, but even that proved too intense with the requirement of being "on" to give lectures and then work one-on-one with students. I would come home and fall asleep at six o'clock. My family called me Rip Van Winkle. Anyone who has chronic illness will understand you lead a secret life, arranging your business hours around rest opportunities and finding excuses for missing weddings or other social events.

When I was working as a journalist, an editor phoned, offering me a lucrative writing assignment that required flying to London to cover a major two-day media event. I was too embarrassed to say crossing the Atlantic twice in three days would exhaust me for weeks. So I chirped, "sure" into the phone before I realized what I had gotten myself into.

There would be endless standing around and walking. Sensible shoes wouldn't cut it. How would I endure standing on my feet for two days? Could I fortify myself with Darvocet for the headaches and caffeine to keep me going? That was as far as I got with the plan. The next night, standing in the departure line at Virgin Airlines, I began counting the hours until I would be back home, lying on my own living room couch.

My first day in London, I woke up in the hotel room, walked into the bathroom and promptly broke my toe by stubbing it on the toilet. I saw stars from the pain. Alone, lying on the bathroom floor, nausea swept over me for ten minutes until I composed myself. The hotel called a doctor who bandaged me up and ordered, "Stay off your feet."

But the temporary physical setback provided surprising advantages. When I went to press gatherings, I was given preference. Walking around with a big, bandaged toe meant I got to sit while the other reporters had to stand. The sore toe gave me an adrenalin surge and made me feisty. When I shouted out questions at the press conference, I always got answers while the burly and pushy types were ignored. One reporter resented this and complained that "Toe Girl" was getting more questions answered than any of the others. My big bandaged toe had turned what I thought would be a sow's ear into a silk purse.

Brain Fog Alert

A few years later, I complained to several doctors that I felt "underwater." The doctors called this condition "brain fog." One doctor told me, "There are things worse than brain fog." Easy for him to say. This frustrating mental impairment was worse than the headaches or fatigue, because thinking was the only thing I had been trained to do. I used to be able to think privately between naps. If I couldn't think straight, I couldn't write. My brain fog caused several friends to yelp when I drove unaware through red traffic lights. I got so many traffic tickets, the state revoked my license and mandated me to attend bad drivers' school.

Even now, when I read my own story it seems unbelievable, but one day from my pre-iodine days reminds me how bad brain fog can get.

I had made an appointment with a respected integrative physician in New York. The day of the appointment I allowed extra time because, as anyone with brain fog knows, you tend to get lost. I was living in the city at the time, and all I needed to do was take the subway straight downtown from the Upper West Side to Midtown. A no brainer. Still, I allowed a full hour extra time. I dressed carefully in a blazer and slacks, applied lipstick and headed out of my apartment building for the half-block walk to the subway. What could go wrong? As I descended the subway steps, I looked down to the bottom of my carefully picked outfit. A pair of fuzzy pink slippers peeked out. Embarrassed, I turned around and returned to my apartment for actual shoes.

Once more, I headed for the subway for the train downtown. I still had plenty of time until my appointment, so I stopped in a luncheonette for a sandwich. But when lunch arrived, I couldn't pay for it because I had forgotten my wallet. The waitress brushed off my second embarrassment of the day, telling me I could pay the next time I came in. I was relieved but my confidence was damaged. If I couldn't get to the doctor's office without two screw-ups, how was I going to find my way home?

I entered the midtown office building and took the elevator up to the office. I checked in with the receptionist and headed for the restroom for a bathroom break. At least I had arrived early. I applied lipstick again and primped, ready to make a good appearance, hoping not to look as goofy as I felt. When I returned to the full waiting room, a white-haired man of about eighty looked at me with alarm.

"Miss," he said, "you have a hanger in your jacket." All eyes turned.

Confused, I thought he meant I had left a dry cleaning tag dangling. I reached up and felt for the back of the jacket collar. Oh, no.

It wasn't a tag. The elderly man was right. A wooden clothes hanger poked from under my blazer. How could I have spent over an hour walking through New York City wearing a jacket with a hanger still attached? My face went red. This signified a new low. I removed my jacket and placed the hanger on the office coat rack. I tried to assume the demeanor of a normal person as I thanked the man and took my seat. But a sinking feeling came over me. What next? At least I wouldn't struggle to explain to the doctor what I meant by "brain fog." I would just describe my day so far.

I didn't know what to try next. My brain didn't have the juice to figure out a strategy. Life decided for me.

Chapter Two

Things Worse Than Brain Fog

Science is the belief in the ignorance of experts.

—Richard P. Feynman

I was diagnosed with breast cancer.

After years of cystic breasts and countless needle biopsies that turned out benign, the last one finally came up positive for cancer. Crap! Now I could not keep impersonating a healthy person. I had to surrender to the fact that my health was out of control. All I could do was put one foot in front of the other. Somebody just had to tell me how and point me in the right direction. Surrendering wasn't as easy as it sounded. Who exactly do I surrender to? I remember hearing about enemy combatants during the Gulf War who wandered around the desert for days looking for someone to surrender to. Surrender implies your struggles will end if you can just find the right person to give up to, no questions asked. That was me.

They Must Know What They Are Doing

Cancer ... A life threatening disease. As in, you can die from that. Fear for your life can make you suspend all questioning and toddle behind the nearest authority figure.

Fear can make you jump onto the first available treatment conveyor belt and plod through the steps assigned to you, no questions asked. Worse, fear can make you believe in the six most dangerous words in the English language: *They must know what they're doing.* Those six words sustained me for about a month.

Got cancer? Step one. Find a well-known doctor at a major Metropolitan hospital. Done. Dr. B. was smart, kind, personable, detail-oriented and open to my endless questions. You would think this partnership between patient and doctor would work out great, right? Well, no and yes. My relationship with the famous surgeon worked out fine right up to the point when she lied to me ... She then mislead me.

To be fair, this arrangement wasn't entirely her fault because it was her job to practice what they call "standard of care" medicine. She was professionally required to follow "treatment guidelines" set up by a specific breast cancer treatment committee. But I didn't know this information at the time. I didn't know the right questions to ask. I had zero context for even asking questions or how to challenge the information she gave me. I had no idea what "survival value" meant.

That was the bad news.

The good news: adrenaline cleared the brain fog, and my determination surged. A light bulb went off. I realized that if the most charming, forthcoming surgeon in the world can legally deceive me, I better find another source of information on breast cancer. My month of surrendering to the powers of a major metropolitan hospital was not as rewarding as I anticipated. I needed to get back in shape and start digging. I needed to study up on how they make recommendations. Where do they get this stuff? Where do they keep the evidence? I needed to read up on the official, so-called, "Breast Cancer Treatment Guidelines."

I no longer had my magic yellow shovel but I knew the principle was the same. Dig. Get the manual. Learn the rules of the game. Talk to anyone and everyone. An editor who mentored me once said, "Sometimes you just have to talk to people until they tell you to go away." He also advised me to always carry a visible notebook and pen. Carrying a notebook makes people talk longer. Why is that? Maybe it gives the person you're talking to the impression they haven't finished. From there on, brandishing my notebook became my best weapon against cancer.

It took me a lot of time and a lot of fact-checking, but I learned how the breast cancer information industry works. I found kindred spirits, and we researched together.

I learned how rare true information scrutiny was in the medical field. I also learned it is considered disrespectful, even treasonous, not to take an oncologist's word for anything.

In many online breast cancer groups, members get upset when you question any authority's position. When patients invest in that authority, they don't want to see their investment devalued or diminished by questioning.

Credentials create a certain momentum of confidence that resists scrutiny. "Questioning behavior" is seen as resistance to authority, when in fact authorities should welcome the opportunity to display the authoritativeness of their learning if that learning is sound.

The specific disease is the grand refuge of the weak, uncultured, unstable minds, such as now rule in the medical profession.

—Florence Nightingale 1820–1910

Chapter Three

Breast Cancer Research
Leads to Iodine

*Healing is a matter of time, but it is sometimes
also a matter of opportunity.*

—Hippocrates

Most surgeons go along with the official Guidelines, thinking those doctors who went before them must be paying attention and know what they were doing because, after all, they're on the Guidelines Committee. Like the rest of us, doctors also have a tendency to believe those terrible six words about the medical system: *They must know what they're doing.* At a local cancer conference, I asked a question of the doctor who served as Director of Breast Cancer Services at one of country's major cancer hospitals.

"Does radiation therapy increase overall survival in breast cancer patients?"
I asked this question because I had researched the medical literature and already knew the answer, which was, *No.* I was testing him to see if his information was reliable.

His answer: "Radiation must increase survival because we do it at our hospital."

I wanted to yell, *Don't you see the flawed logic in that answer? Whatever you do must be right because you do it?* But I stood silent in the back of the audience knowing I had just witnessed one of the most bizarre, arrogant moments in medical history. And nobody screamed, not even me. We were too stunned.

Thus, I began my mission as breast cancer information activist. I was not going to keep the real evidence a secret. The evidence is available to everybody online in the National Library of Medicine. Medical information isn't locked in a silver trunk anymore, where only the privileged few can access it. Is looking up studies an alternative practice? Only if you consider locating and disclosing peer review evidence subversive!

> *I was trained never to share the deeper levels of my thinking with patients. And when I took the Hippocratic Oath in 1989, I swore to keep my medical knowledge secret. So until quite recently, becoming a knowledgeable, involved and medically competent participant in one's medical care was simply not permitted. And there is a good deal of physician resistance, resentment, and denial to the inescapable fact that the Internet is helping patients become better informed, more responsible, and more medically competent.*
> —Alan Greene, MD, Clinical Professor of Pediatrics
> Stanford, E-patients White Paper

Breast Cancer Choices

I founded a nonprofit organization called Breast Cancer Choices, Inc. At our website, *www.BreastCancerChoices.org*, you can see our organization specializes in scrutinizing the available information about breast cancer. Our mission contains three goals: disclosure,

disclosure, disclosure. I didn't become a breast cancer information activist because I had time on my hands. I had no choice. Doing my own detective work was the only other option, once my surrender strategy didn't work out.

I trained myself to scrutinize studies for breast cancer treatments and therapies because I didn't know any other way of getting the information. My doctors didn't seem to be looking at the primary literature. When I asked my oncologist for the studies, she said she'd have to ask somebody where they were.

If she had actually read the primary literature, she would know that the evidence didn't fit with the official Guidelines.

Oncologists and surgeons were too busy following the committee-generated Guidelines to verify if they were evidence-based or not. All you need to do is look it up and you will see that in breast cancer, what they refer to as evidence-based medicine is *not* evidence based. It's *consensus-based*. Big difference. Life-altering difference. *Evidence-based* medicine means survival was extended within a group of studied people. *Consensus–based* medicine means a bunch of doctors think a treatment is a good idea. Honest. Go ahead—do a fact-check on this.

Again, a physical setback in my life turned out to have a silver lining. This time it wasn't breaking my big toe that saved me at a press conference; it was breast cancer, forcing me to dig deeper and not surrender to the status quo. The thrill of uncovering hidden information is an emotion as powerful as any gateway drug. I was hooked and could not turn back.

Digging into breast cancer research lead me to iodine. I didn't think I could ever be more passionate about anything than I was about the dubious world of cancer treatment. But then, one fall day, an accidental meeting changed all that.

Let me tell you how this scenario not only revived my obsession with the sea, but ignited a passion to spread the word about seaweed and iodine to whoever will listen.

In 2005, Sherri Tenpenny, D.O., introduced herself to me at The American College for the Advancement of Medicine (ACAM) conference and asked if I had heard anything about using iodine for the breast. I replied I was only aware of Ghent and Eskin's work on iodine helping fibrocystic (benign) breast disease.

Benign disease was, after all, a totally different condition than malignant disease. *Right?*

I had been a breast cancer information activist for many years, going to all the conferences, networking with the most progressive doctors. Certainly if iodine was good for breast cancer, I would have heard about it. *Right?*

Wrong, wrong, wrong!

Only because I respected Dr. Tenpenny so much as a famous vaccine educator, did I consider her suggestion to investigate iodine more. When I returned home, I Googled "iodine breast" and there were very few hits. So I searched the National Library of Medicine Database known as Pubmed. I found researchers in at least five countries had made major connections between breast tumors and iodine deficiency. The research went back almost 50 years. I was humbled and confused. Still, the same arrogant phrase played in a loop in my head. I had studied breast cancer and every conceivable approach for more than a decade. *I would have heard about iodine if it had anything to do with breast cancer.*

I gave myself two weeks to read the full articles of the iodine research and see what I could discover. Then I had to locate some of the papers and books in their bibliographies, so I budgeted another month of time to research. Then another month. I couldn't understand how the link between iodine and breast disease had been logged into The National Library of Medicine for 50 years and never made it into sources I would know.

Why didn't the research scientists present their findings at medical conferences? I was tempted to psychologize that perhaps scientists were shyer than the rest of us, or they didn't want to be accused by their peers of overstating the significance of their findings.

I needed more intellectual confidence. I hadn't yet heard of Dr. Guy Abraham ... or, that there had been a virtual moratorium on iodine research for the last 50 years. I was still reasoning like a conventional person and didn't understand what Dr. David Brownstein calls the "Alice in Wonderland" part of contemporary medicine.

As an independent scholar, I practice information investigation, not medicine.

I've discovered since, that not all research is online. You need to go out into the real world. I began to dig up old pharmacy ledgers. I bid on old iodine "junk" at auctions; found 100 year-old veterinary pamphlets on putting iodine in livestock feed; located a 1950s pamphlet on how to cure nymphomania by prescribing an anti-iodine drug.

Now my office stands are piled with old iodine medical books stacked against the walls. Research papers bulge from file cabinets. My iodine investigation expanded far out from the official medical literature and into the disciplines of geology, anthropology, neurology and archeology. This may be an un-orthodox way of doing research, but I didn't have to account to the limitations of a consensus-driven, peer-review committee, and I didn't have a medical license to lose. As an independent scholar, I practice information investigation, not medicine. So I could follow the iodine research wherever the investigation took me and report the truth.

Besides investigating medical and non-medical scholarship, I found I could reconstruct the nineteenth and twentieth century iodine use by locating actual iodine artifacts through collectors selling antique medical items. In a lay effort at the forensic anthropology of iodine, Breast Cancer Choices managed to collect a Civil War iodine canteen, iodine inhalation devices, various syphilis formulas, a 50 year-old iodine locket from the British Red Cross and ointments for breast cysts, to name a few. We even located a can of iodine powder that dates back to when Van Gogh raved to his brother how great iodine was for syphilis! If Dr. Tenpenny had not sent me on the two week research project that lasted eight years, I would not have ended up with an office that smells like medicine. I wouldn't have learned that iodine and seaweed can be documented as the oldest traditional medicine or that a lost medical heirloom has finally been found .

Launcher of the Iodine Movement

In 2005, I was still limited to reviewing the published medical literature. Dr. Guy Abraham, a retired professor of obstetrics, gynecology and endocrinology at UCLA School of Medicine, had published material challenging what is known as the "Wolff-Chaikoff Effect," a relatively new (1961), but text book-accepted, theory about the "dangers of iodine." One of his research partners, Dr. Jorge Flechas, was scheduled to speak on iodine at a conference in Los Angeles.

Without hesitation, I crossed the country to hear him speak and to introduce myself. My colleagues from the cancer activist community also attended the iodine talk and were as intrigued as I was by his compelling information and broad comprehension of iodine. Dr. Flechas' presentation was voted the best speech at the conference by an informal poll done afterward. He distributed detailed materials on Dr. Abraham's Iodine Project and the new thinking about iodine. What an adventure! What a find!

Visit Dr. Flechas' website at *http://cypress.he.net/*.

When I returned to the East Coast, I excitedly reported the Abraham-Brownstein-Flechas Iodine Project information to my online breast cancer group. What do you think happened? They responded the same way I did when Dr. Tenpenny introduced iodine as a breast therapy to me a year earlier.

"Iodine?

Iodine and breast cancer?

Lynne, are you nuts?"

So I engaged some research partners and we persevered. We began taking iodine ourselves, first the traditional Lugol's Iodine Solution which had been used for over 175 years, then a new product, a Lugol's Iodine tablet called Iodoral. I started with one 12.5 mg tablet. I didn't notice any change. After a few months, I decided to take the 24 hour urine Iodine Loading Test to measure my baseline iodine levels.

The test procedure requires taking 50 mg of Iodoral in the morning and then collecting urine for 24 hours to see how much of the 50 mg is absorbed and how much is excreted.

Within two hours of taking the 50 mg of Iodoral, I got a sensation some of us call "the boing." My brain cleared as if the dusty unused rooms of my brain suddenly got oxygen. My thoughts grew

sharper edges. I felt a burst of energy, thought faster and felt smarter even doing everyday math. I remember getting impatient with a store clerk because he couldn't compute three times thirty times two in his mind. After several tries, he pulled out a calculator. Before iodine I wouldn't have even noticed.

Some other iodine takers have reported this instant effect. Dr. William Shevin reported occasionally seeing this phenomenon in his own practice when he spoke at the first Iodine Conference in 2007. He said, "Those patients are so iodine deficient, they are going on fumes." Dr. Shevin also showed a video of a patient describing his new mental clarity on iodine supplementation. It was like to turning the dial of radio until you get the absolute clearest reception from a channel.

Nobody can explain the physiology of the "boing" reaction with any certainty. Is it the thyroid? Neurologists trained in iodine deficiency would probably explain the intellectual zap as entirely neurological. At this point, nobody knows!

Bottom line: After I raised my Iodoral dosage, my brain not only snapped to attention, my weight normalized, my skin lost its lifelong dryness and several mysterious cysts disappeared. My cold feet were now warm. I only get a headache now if I stretch wrong. The orange Darvocet vial, my constant companion for years, now rests in the local landfill.

Other Iodine Leaders Appear and the Revolution Ignites

A small body of determined spirits fired by an unquenchable faith in their mission can alter the course of history.
—Mahatma Ghandi

Soon after, we at Breast Cancer Choices met Zoe Alexander, a retired professor who started an online group to discuss iodine usage by patients. As a scholar, she started an additional group just for iodine researchers. When the online file space became overloaded, Zoe created a comprehensive, scholarly website, *Iodine4Health.com*, now revived as IodineResearch.com where she compiled every iodine resource she could find. With the true spirit of grass roots innovation, the website launched on an independent server by fellow iodine activists, Lynn Razaitis and Curt Smith. *IodineResearch.com*

Other groups started investigating iodine, finding even more research and compared notes on supplementing iodine. Testimonials began coming forth. Detoxification problems found solutions. The Curezone Iodine Forum, which as of this printing, continues to be led by two of its three original founders, Laura "Wombat" Olsson and Steve "Trapper" Wilson, became hugely active and well-respected as an experimental iodine users group. Visit the forum at *http://curezone.com/forums/f.asp?f=815.*

The Curezone Iodiners were viciously attacked when they started. Their attackers predicted they would all end up in the hospital or morgue from taking iodine. Now their attackers have mysteriously disappeared and the group is thriving.

The Iodine Curezoners took nothing on face value and established a reputation for fact-checking and mining of historical uses of iodine. The Curezoners were infected with the research bug acquired from the Dr. Abraham research. It was known as *the Abraham Effect*, a behavior characterized by the obsession to research and document the wealth of historical uses of iodine.

The Curezone Iodine Forum logged over ten million hits, making it a testament to the power of grassroots medicine. Laura Olsson and Steve Wilson have become so knowledgeable about iodine they have created their own unique and well-respected iodine products.

Chapter Four

Bromine—
A Cause for Iodine Deficiency

Research is formalized curiosity.
It is poking and prying with a purpose.

—Zora Neale Huston

Within a few years, the success of the iodine users within the online groups went viral. Thyroid and fibromyalgia groups took up the iodine cause. Mothering groups tried it and reported success. Gradually more and more nutrition groups could not argue with the success so many experienced. Meanwhile in the years since my accidental meeting with Dr. Tenpenny, I've dug deeper with my research and uncovered an alarming pattern.

We've become iodine deficient since the 1970s because the anti-iodine bromine has purged iodine from our bodies!

Breast cancer rates have risen since the 1970s as iodine consumption decreased and anti-iodine bromine exposure increased. I also looked at the Department of Defense statistics on bromide exposure in Gulf War veterans. The bromism symptoms seem to parallel other exposures, especially the ubiquitous brominated fire retardants that we sleep on every night and sit on every day in furniture. I created a Powerpoint presentation titled *The Perfect Storm Theory of Breast Cancer* (see Chapter 18: *The Perfect Storm of Breast Cancer*) which explores this phenomenon.

It became clear that we aren't just iodine deficient because we don't eat enough eggs or seafood. We've become iodine deficient since the 1970s because the iodine-blocking element bromine has purged iodine from our bodies. *The Bromide Dominance theory,* explained in Appendix B in *The Iodine Crisis,* may account for why more people are sick, IQs are dropping while thyroid and other diseases continue to worsen. Obesity may not have to do with overeating as much as a bromine-caused metabolic slow-down that causes weight gain.

Bromine, the Evil "Holy Grail" of Iodine Deficiency

Yes, the bromine-saturated environment can make you both fat and stupid.

Below are six points targeting the dangers of our bromine-saturated environment and the need for supplementing iodine as compensation. Consider these points a call to action.

1. Bromine fire retardant poisoning increases every year and takes years to reverse, making bromide the toxic equivalent to Global Warming.
2. Bromide pesticides and fire retardants will wind up being the new DDT, a pesticide banned in 1972, is still present in the breast tissue of women born later than that date.
3. If the underlying cause of thyroid, breast and other hormone-driven diseases is iodine deficiency, then bromide dominance is the underlying cause of that deficiency.

Figure 1
The Underlying Cause of the Underlying Cause?

Bromide Dominance, underlying cause of iodine deficiency 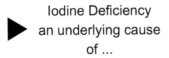 Iodine Deficiency an underlying cause of ... 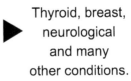 Thyroid, breast, neurological and many other conditions.

4. Iodine is the biochemical "antidote" for toxic bromine but it takes time. Bromine is a persistent chemical bully. Like any bully, it has to be outflanked, outnumbered and outwitted. The right dosage of iodine is your ally.
5. Bromine toxicity is too important to leave to the slow bureaucratic systems of policy making. We have to teach ourselves and each other.
6. I share the goals of the Grass Roots Iodine Movement trailblazers. Let's spread the iodine information far and wide, to our families, our neighbors and the world.

Iodine Fast Stats

The term "Iodine" was Googled 1,220,000 times during the month of September, 2012.

- The World Health Organization cites iodine deficiency as the most preventable cause of mental retardation. Iodine deficiency doesn't just occur in poor countries. If babies are not born with profound intelligent defects, even with mild iodine deficiencies, many babies are significantly less smart than they could be. Also note that autism rates are rising significantly.

- Iodine consumption has decreased 50 percent since the 1970s.
- Iodine deficiency diseases of the breast, prostate and thyroid, have increased during that time.
- Thyroid cancer rates rose 182 percent between 1975 and 2005.
- Breast Cancer has risen from 1 in 23 to 1 in 7-8 since the 1970s.
- Iodine deficiency is higher every time the government agency measures it.
- Iodine deficiency in pregnant women is producing less intelligent children.

Part 2

Frequently Asked Questions (FAQ)

Disclaimer: *The iodine referred to throughout* **The Iodine Crisis** *does not refer to Tincture of Iodine you may find in your medicine chest. Do not take iodine without consulting an Iodine Literate Practitioner and your personal licensed health professional. The information in this book is not intended to replace the relationship with your health professional. Neither the author nor publisher of this book takes responsibility for any consequences for any health strategy published in this book. The author reports the information as a journalist, not a doctor. The information below is the result of the shared patient-to-patient research and should not be construed as medical advice.*

Since most readers of this book are not chemists, consider the terms iodine and iodide interchangeable unless the difference is relevant to the discussion such as the iodide in iodized salt.

Similarly, the reader should consider the terms bromine and bromide interchangeable; the power of any bromine-related chemical to inhibit iodine is illustrated and discussed.

List of Frequently Asked Questions

Chapter Five

FAQ 1
Why Does Your Body Need Iodine?

What is iodine?

Iodine is an essential micro-nutrient. This means it is needed in small amounts by every cell in the body. Iodine can be very powerful and our bodies have built in compensation mechanisms to conserve it. That's the good news.

Then there is the bad news. Iodine deficiency has become a public health crisis because it's so vulnerable to displacement by environmental toxins such as bromide, pesticides and food additives. That's exactly what's causing the iodine deficiency. Bromine fire retardants surround us. Introduced in the 1970s, they have accumulated in our homes, cars and work places. Iodine as a food fortifier was removed from flour around the same time, contributing to the iodine deficiency that has grown to epidemic proportions.

Is nutritional iodine the same as the iodine in the medicine cabinet?

Tincture of Iodine is made with alcohol for use as a topical antiseptic. This alcohol form of iodine is not made for oral consumption and is usually marked with a skull and cross bones signifying a poison. The main form of iodine used for the supplementation iodine we consume as a supplement is Lugol's Iodine Solution or Lugol's in tablet form (Iodoral™). Other formulations are manufactured but *The Iodine Crisis* speaks only to the Lugol's formulation.

Why has iodine become big news now?

Because some brilliant doctors fact-checked the medical literature, then refuted the recent myth that iodine supplementation was toxic. They went back in history to when iodine was a universally used medicine and reported the information. The double whammy came when tens of thousands of medical consumers tried supplementing iodine and began reporting success stories on the Internet. The Grass Roots Iodine Movement was born! Patient success, research and supplementation reports continue to fuel interest in iodine.

Is iodine a prescription item?

Iodine is available as a nutritional supplement just as any vitamin or mineral.

How was iodine used in the past?

From medical records in 1906, iodine was considered The Universal Medicine" and used to treat:

Goiter
Atherosclerosis
Syphilis
Uterine fibroids
Mercury, lead and arsenic poisoning
Swollen glands
Prostatic hypertrophy
Scarlet fever

Bronchitis and pneumonia
Obesity
Depression
Breast pain
Eczema
Genito-urinary diseases
Malaria
Ovarian cysts
"Rheumatism"
Gastralgia
Tonsilitis
Cough

Figure 2
The 1899 Merck Manual Was the
World's Best-selling Medical Textbook

MERCK'S 1899 MANUAL.

PART FIRST.

THE MATERIA MEDICA,

As in Actual Use To-day by American Physicians.

As far back as 1899, the world's best-selling medical text-book, the Merck Manual, cited iodine as the most used substance for tumors. But Iodine's therapeutic range goes much broader. In Chapter 14: *The Buried History of Iodine*, I explain how seaweed-based medicine and iodine goes back 15,000 years. But the "Golden Age of Iodine" spanned the last half of the 1800s and into the first half of the 1900s.

Don't I get enough iodine in iodized salt?

The notion that refined iodized salt is sufficient is the most dangerous misconception about iodine. From the time iodized salt leaves the factory until it gets on grocery store shelves, half of the original iodide content is lost. Because once iodized salt is opened in your home, the iodine "sublimes" or escapes into the air in varying degrees, depending on humidity. After all that, when ingested, only 10 percent of the iodine in salt is absorbable. Then, after all that, again, women should be concerned that the "iodine" in salt is actually iodide. Iodine is preferred by the breasts, thus a combination of iodine and iodide is generally used. Also, did I mention that cooking destroys iodine? Iodized Salt researchers, Dasgupta, et al, report on the problems of iodized salt in *Iodine Nutrition: Iodine Content of Salt in the United States.*

Did I mention that common refined sodium chloride is devoid of any naturally occurring minerals contained in nutritious un-refined salt such as Celtic Sea Salt?

So—short answer: No, you can't get enough iodine from iodized salt because you can't be sure if you're actually getting iodine—how much or what kind. The "Iodized Salt Scam" is discussed in Chapter 8. *How Often Should I Take Iodine?*, When ingested, only 10 percent of the iodine in salt is absorbable.

I eat a lot of fish so I probably don't need iodine, right?

If you eat four pounds of ocean fish every day, *bon appetit!* Most iodine literate practitioners would say you probably don't have to worry about iodine, just the mercury in four pounds of fish.

Is iodine safe to supplement?

Iodine is safe when the right product is taken as directed under the supervision of an Iodine Literate Practitioner.

If iodine has been around so long, why aren't people using it medically anymore?

When patent antibiotics such as penicillin came into use after World War II, Iodine was considered "old-fashioned," a cardinal sin in the medical community. Gradually, its traditional properties, other than use as an antiseptic became virtually unknown. But the fatal blow came when an influential medical paper mistakenly claimed iodine was dangerous. A moratorium on iodine use began and iodine's use and its benefits gradually disappeared except for antiseptic purposes. The mistake in one influential paper purged the benefits of iodine for two generations of Medical School students. The effect of this research paper is discussed in detail in the Chapters 16, *Who Stole Iodine from my Medicine?* and Chapter 17, *Who Stole Iodine from my Food?*

What is iodine deficiency?

There are various technical definitions of iodine "deficiency" and "sufficiency" and much disagreement among health professionals. An Iodine Literate Practitioner would describe a patient as iodine deficient based on a combination of symptoms and/or the Iodine Loading Test.

But isn't the iodine RDA for adults 150 mcg which I get in my multivitamin?

The RDA appears to be calculated from how much iodine the thyroid needs to avoid goiter. The requirements of the other organs aren't factored into the number. Additionally, the effect of iodine-blocking polluters was never considered when 150 mcg was established.

What are the iodine deficiency symptoms?

Often we don't know which symptoms *are* iodine deficiency-related until they disappear after taking iodine. Veteran iodine takers report they feel increasing improvement as the months and years go on. Conditions such as psoriasis, coldness and even testicular cysts have disappeared in people using iodine for other reasons.

Originally, we thought iodine must be helping the thyroid because that was the main gland known for storing iodine. Since then, if someone's hearing improves, for example, we think iodine is helping the neurological system. Since every cell in the body contains iodine, we can't know the mechanism of action. The only way to define what makes an iodine deficiency is by listing what symptoms iodine has benefited.

In developing countries, iodine deficiency is the leading cause of goiter and mental retardation. In my own experience as well as the experience of many other iodine-takers, even the average person experiences a boost in perception and the ability to make calculations.

A partial list of conditions we've seen that are helped by iodine:

Allergies
Brain fog
Dry skin
Cysts and nodules
Fatigue
Thyroid problems
Ovarian problems
Cognitive problems (unclear thinking)
Menstrual irregularities
Weight gain
Breast pain/ fibrocystic breast disease
Feeling cold
Gum infection
Psoriasis

Type 2 Diabetes
Hair thinning
Puffy face
Fertility problems
Depression
Heart arrhythmia
Blood pressure
Cholesterol
Scars
Infections
Genital Herpes
Miscarriage
Fibromyalgia
Hearing loss
Prostate disease
Lung conditions
Constipation
Fertility (in women)
Vaginal infections
Eye problems
Neck pain
GERD
Excema
Resistance to colds and virus
Increased sex drive
Increased erections and semen when applied to the testicles

Can I get enough iodine from dried seaweed or seaweed supplement products?

1. There's a danger that the seaweed may have picked up arsenic, heavy metals, oil spill dispersants, radiation or other contaminants from our now-polluted seawater. Also, you never know how much iodine you're getting in

such items as kelp tablets or what the ingredients used as tablet filler and binders do. Seaweed loses much of its iodine content after harvesting, so after being reprocessed into tablets, and stockpiled in a warehouse for months, do you really know what you're taking?

2. The Fukushima Japanese nuclear reactor explosion seems to have contaminated much of the world's seaweed. This nuclear contamination has been virtually ignored outside Japan. Although, according to *The Maritime Executive* publication, The Institute for Radiological Protection and Nuclear Safety reported that the Fukushima disaster produced the world's worst nuclear sea pollution. Also, we've almost forgotten about the oil spills in the US Gulf that have migrated far out and the dispersants used to dissolve the oil present additional sea life contamination problems. We don't know how long crops of seaweed remain contaminated.

How do I know if I'm iodine deficient?

The most definitive way to diagnose iodine deficiency is to be evaluated by an Iodine Literate Practitioner. The results of taking the Iodine Loading Test is used to get a baseline to determine how much iodine is saturated in the tissues.

What makes an Iodine Literate Practitioner?

Breast Cancer Choices and the major iodine patient-to-patient online groups customarily define an Iodine Literate Practitioner as someone who has read all the writings of the Iodine Project initiated by A. Guy Abraham, MD, David Brownstein, MD, and Jorge Flechas, MD.

Additionally, an Iodine Literate Practitioner is conversant with the book, *Iodine: Why You Need It: Why You Can't Live Without It*, fourth edition, by David Brownstein, MD. These works explain the comprehensive context of iodine therapy and how the 50 mg dose was arrived at. An Iodine Literate Practitioner will be familiar with the necessity of the companion nutrients and will never recommend seaweed as a substitute for iodine.

If a practitioner routinely prescribes for adults, an amount of iodine under 50 mg; does not know why each of the companion nutrients is used (including selenium for Hashimoto's Thyroiditis); is unfamiliar with salt loading, auto-immune disease treatment or interpreting the idiosyncrasies of iodine patient TSH test reports; then Breast Cancer Choices does not recommend them as iodine literate. Many doctors claim they are iodine literate but recommend kelp or very weak iodine products. Check with the patient-to-patient iodine groups online to make sure you are using a time-tested product or ask an experienced practitioner.

Please check the website *www.BreastCancerChoices.org/IPrac titioners* which is updated frequently. The website does not include every practitioner using iodine since more prescribe iodine every day.

I heard there is a quick "patch test" to see if you are iodine deficient. What is that test and how accurate is it?

The so-called iodine patch test refers to painting a two inch square of tincture of iodine or Lugol's Iodine on the body and watching to see how long the orange square takes to fade. Theoretically, the quicker the orange fades, the hungrier your body is for iodine. However, so many variables exist in human skin, that the test cannot be considered reliable or conclusive.

Additionally:

1. The body may be dehydrated on that day.
2. The skin may be more or less iodine deficient than, say, the ovaries.

3. The gold standard in the Iodine Movement is to assess iodine deficiency with the 24 hour Iodine Loading Test.

Where do I get the Iodine Loading Test?

Ask your doctor for a lab she prefers or look in **The Iodine Loading Test** section in Part 4, *Resources,* of this book. Patients can order this test without a prescription.

Do vegetarians need iodine?

Yes, especially if they are not eating seaweed five times per day or in the quantities the average resident of Japan consumes. As mentioned earlier, eating seaweeds is a risky way to consume iodine, and it loses iodine rapidly after harvesting.

Can everybody take iodine?

In seven years, I've only met a handful people who said they could not tolerate iodine. Some gave up quickly after getting a rash, brain fog or fatigue and did not do the salt loading protocol. Others have experienced other problems and are still working to resolve those issues. And still others swear iodine doesn't agree with them. Iodine is necessary to stay alive and is already in the tissue of every human being, so the people who can't tolerate iodine need an experienced practitioner to investigate why supplementation is causing problems.

If you are allergic to the iodine contrast dyes in scans, are you allergic to iodine?

The radioactive iodine in medical scans is an entirely different substance from the iodine in iodine supplements. The Iodine doctors have reported that only if you are allergic to iodized salt will you be allergic to iodine.

I'm allergic to shellfish. Can I take iodine?

Most people who are allergic to shellfish can take iodine supplements. Shellfish contains a protein which is a common allergen. Again, the Iodine Literate Practitioners find that only people allergic to iodized salt may be allergic to iodine supplementation.

Is iodine just another thing that's "good for me?" It sounds too good to be true.

Iodine is a universal nutrient in that it regulates hormones and metabolism, enhances brain development and function as well as detoxifies toxic halogens and heavy metals. Iodine works as an "adaptogen," that is, it helps strengthen the body's ability to adapt to and compensate for physical disruptions.

If you think iodine is just another nutrient, read the diverse success stories in this book and decide for yourself.

Iodine Success Stories

The iodine success stories reported throughout this book established an unexpected milestone in my iodine journey. Over the years, people had emailed me their successes and thanked me for publishing the iodine information on the website. Many other success stories were recorded by the Curezone Forum and Yahoo Iodine Group. But I had never asked for stories until the final stages of writing this book. I only expected to document a record of iodine supplementers. But something intensely powerful happened. When I sent out three emails to different groups, people opened up their hearts to me and shared their struggles and successes. It changed many lives, from allergies, to debilitating fatigue, to being able to get out of bed and go to work. Others found iodine stopped horrible menstrual problems. Still others found their prostates became healthy and their libidos returned. The generous outpouring of those who have suffered moved me in ways I'm still trying to process. I thank them all.

41

I discovered that people who have recovered from many years of stoicism want to tell their stories. They want to offer their experience in the chance that someone else will benefit as much as they did. Many of us sound like evangelists because the course of our lives was transformed. Iodine is not a panacea, but it has mysteriously and powerfully altered who we are as individuals and family members. We want to do something with the good fortune we have received. We want to "pay it forward" as the saying goes.

Meet Kim: Her sense of well-being returned, and her hair loss stopped.

Iodine changed my life.

I was searching for "perfect health" and the answer was iodine. I started taking iodine in April, 2011. At the time, I didn't know about Iodoral so I found a compounding pharmacy willing to make Lugol's iodine for me. I had iodine-related bromide symptoms right away on one drop. At the time I had joined a learn-to-run group, and I remember the symptoms showing strongly when I tried to run. My nose dripped, I couldn't run very far without being exhausted, and I was depressed and having dark thoughts.

I tend to be quite brave about plowing through detox symptoms. I understand natural healing and what occurs, so despite the anxiety, depression and dark thoughts, I kept going. I did a lot of salt loading that helped immensely. My urine had a strange smell.

I had a lot of clashes with my mother. I feel badly about it now but healing takes place from the head down. I obviously had some suppressed anger and she was the one I took it out on.

I gave up using conventional deodorant and switched to a natural one. Always "needing" deodorant, when I switched, I went through a time period of heavy body odor. I remember one day a friend looking at me, wondering why I smelled so bad. I wish I had said, "Oh sorry, I know I stink, I am detoxing," but I didn't. I am thrilled to say, that period has passed and I barely need deodorant now. Seriously! I hardly need it!

From the very beginning, my thyroid felt swollen and I was always looking in the mirror to see if it looked strange. I don't think it did but I was definitely worried. The muscles around my jaw and my shoulders felt tight. I was grinding my teeth. My skin took on a white, translucent look and my nails shone! Today I get complimented often on my "nice tan" even though I haven't been in the sun. I do wonder if the iodine has made my skin a little darker.

As the year progressed, I kept taking a little more and a little more iodine. I found out about Iodoral, and I found it so much easier than the drops. My hair, which had fallen out all my adult life, stopped falling out. I even think my grey hair took on a tinge of colour again.

There were two things I noticed that I am not sure if they were always there, or I just came out of my brain fog and finally noticed them; my tongue was sore and I had quite a few cherry angiomas.

By February, I was able to take four Iodoral (50 mg) without too much trouble. This for me was a miracle. It was a long road to "no detox symptoms" for me. One of the most amazing things was that the chiropractor I had been seeing for years started to say "You are in really good shape." My general aches and pains had definitely disappeared.

At this time, however, I really did feel that my detox pathways (liver, kidneys) had had enough and needed a break. I did gain weight. I was also reading what Dr. Brownstein and Dr. Abraham were saying about lowering the dose after a year. I have two things to say about this time. One was that at the back of my mind, I thought maybe I should go to a higher dose, and two, instead of doing what was advised and lowering the dose to 12.5, I stopped altogether. I can't comment on what I should have done. This was my journey.

I took some time to see an acupuncturist to help with my detox pathways, and at this time, I started feeling "spiritual." I have delved deeper into this and I now meditate daily. The iodine had opened my "third eye" but it took stopping the iodine for me to see that.

I stopped until recently but started back at 50mg of iodine a day with no trouble at all. I have even tried raising the dose to 100mg on and off.

It is my desire to tell others about iodine. I am grateful for this opportunity. I believe that it is a great healer and has the potential to bring joy back into people's lives. Be strong on your journey, you CAN heal.

Meet Marty: Crippling fatigue, depression and a worsening spiral begin to resolve.

Greetings, I am a 31 year old male who has been on Lugol's 2% iodine for the past 33 days.

For most of my life I have had trouble with fatigue and brain fog, but, in hindsight, the signs were obvious because of puberty, It was at that point I developed gynecomastia (breast tissue), bad scalp problems (bloody scabs from the itching), emotionality/ neurotic behavior, poor lower jaw development, poor beard development and much more.

I've been labeled with many different learning and cognitive disabilities by schools and have been called lazy since around age 14 when the fatigue started to get bad. My hair started to fall out at 17, then started to slowly turn white by 21, very notice-able by 25. I have never lived on my own as the fatigue has al-ways crushed any attempts to pursue a serious goal. Since age 17, I've been on many dreaded SSRI [antidepressant] cycles doc-tors prescribe as a band-aid to deeper, more fundamental issues.

About a year ago, after researching something unrelated, it occurred to me that I had some sort of hormone problem which I suspected was hypogonadism rooted in either not enough native testosterone production, or too much phytoestrogens disrupting normal endocrine function. Without health insurance or income, there was no choice but to explore options other than drugs. So I tried many things such as DHEA, and antioxidants such as grape seed extract and indole 3 carbinole (I3C).

Nothing seemed to have an effect on the crippling fatigue, but then I came across the symptoms of hypothyroidism in a book my mother had. It was like reading a personal biography, a notion reinforced when I then started to research personal testimonials online. I came across the idea of taking iodine after reading some articles, on Lugol's 2% and 5%. There were many positive testimonials there, so I went for it.

The first week I was sick a lot, headaches and fatigue, dark thoughts and such. *Only later I learned that salt water and the companion nutrients would have helped that.* Fortunately, my mother had all kinds of vitamin C and magnesium tablets, and I had already been on a multi-vitamin for several months. I started with 12.5 mg of iodine and was up to 50 by the first week. I stayed on 50 mg for a solid 10 days before trying 75 mg, and the increase in energy was quite noticeable.

About a week ago, I started consuming Celtic sea salt and so far it looks like I am gradually getting better. Last week I helped a family member with some construction type work for a good three hours, which is the first time I've been compelled to labor like that for many years. I came back a few days later and helped for three straight days about four hours each, which would have been out of the question just a week or two prior.

There is still some fatigue during the day, especially after I eat, but actually falling asleep from it is becoming increasingly rare. In fact, there were signs of progress even in the first week, as the bloody scabs on my crown went away though there is still some flaking, and the hair shedding has significantly reduced. Today I'll be taking 125 mg to see if the progress continues.

As I said, I have tried many things with depressing results. This is the first time I have noticed any considerable change. I am hopeful (desperate) that this iodine protocol is the first step in turning things around for my health, and maybe soon I will have the strength to work and not have the constant reminder of how emasculating it is not to be independent.

Meet Betty: Diabetes and related stomach problem resolve.

I only started using Lugol's because I had stomach and intestinal bacterial overgrowth (Gastroparesis, a common occurrence with Diabetics where the stomach takes 15 to 20 hours to empty). This causes many symptoms. Lugol's worked very well and took care of the symptoms, and the BONUS was that I no longer need to take my diabetes pills. I've been off them for two weeks now (in 13 years), and my blood sugars are staying within normal levels which didn't happen even WHILE I was taking them. I am very happy, and I want everyone to KNOW what iodine has done for me. I can't tell enough people.

Nice that I can get complacent, huh? One in seven American women will be diagnosed with breast cancer. I'm sure that I will not. I have experienced iodine and companion nutrients dissolving fibrous tissue.

Too bad I didn't know about this five years ago, when my sister-in-law died of breast cancer. She left five children behind.

Chapter Six

FAQ 2
Why Consider
Supplementing Iodine?

Is Iodine a magic bullet?
Iodine is not something that's just "good for you." The effect lies in its profound power to detox, normalize and nourish the cells so they can work optimally. From an evolutionary perspective, Dr. Sebastiano Venturi suggests that iodine in the form of seaweed was probably the first anti-oxidant. Iodine is more of a missing link that helps the body regulate and adapt. That's why it's called "the universal nutrient." But no one should consider iodine a cure-all for anything.

What dosage of iodine is right for me?
Most people determine their dosage by trial and error and with the support of their Iodine Literate Practitioner or with the support of the online Iodine Groups. See The Iodine Supplementation Protocol, in Part 4, *Resources*.

Which kind of Iodine is the best to take?
My family and friends prefer Iodoral, a form of Lugol's Solution compounded in tablet form to protect the stomach. A single 12.5

mg Iodoral tablet contains two different kinds of iodine: 5 mg iodine and 7.5 mg potassium iodide. We also keep a bottle of Lugol's Iodine in the car and in the medicine chest for first aid or digestive problems.

Others prefer the original Lugol's Solution, SSKI, Magnascent or other forms. It's helpful to ask members of the online iodine forums why they prefer one over the other. You will find some iodine "gourmets" out there who combine different iodine formulations.

Since I can only vouch for Iodoral and Lugol's Iodine Solution as effective from personal experience, I can't knowledgeably recommend other formulations. However, I would be hesitant to buy any iodine "formulations" which combine tyrosine or selenium in the same tablet. Many products have sprung up to meet the demand of iodine-savvy consumers. Unfortunately, not all of these products are based on a broad knowledge of iodine metabolism.

How many milligrams of iodine do Lugol's Solution drops contain? How does that compare to Iodoral?

2 drops of Lugol's 5% Solution contain the equivalent of one tablet of Iodoral 12.5 mg. See the **Lugol's Iodine Solution Chart** in the *Resources* section of this book.

Is there a consensus on dosing iodine?

Ask your Iodine Literate Practitioner. The usual goal for adults is to start with 12.5 mg and work up to 50 mg or more if a medical condition is at issue. The experience of many iodine takers has shown that building up the dose gradually helps reduce side effects. It may take some time to find the right dosage. Most people find contacting the online Iodine Groups helpful. Patient-to-patient experts with years of experience will provide information.

Do I take iodine all at once or spread the dosage out through the day?

Most people prefer to take iodine in the morning because of the possibility of iodine causing wakefulness at bedtime. Others spread it out during the day.

If iodine is so good at killing bacteria, won't it kill off the beneficial bacteria in my gut?

Iodine killing off gut bacteria has never been reported. Some scientists think the original source of iodine from seaweed makes it protective as one of the original antioxidants from an evolutionary point of view.

Can I consume Tincture of Iodine instead?

No. Absolutely not! Tincture of Iodine is considered toxic if taken by mouth.

Can I consume Betadine?

No. Absolutely not! Betadine iodine is considered toxic if taken by mouth.

Can I consume Povidone?

No. Absolutely not! Povidone iodine is considered toxic if taken by mouth.

I don't have a thyroid. Does my body need iodine?

Yes. Every cell in the body requires iodine to function, everybody needs iodine.

Where can I buy iodine supplements?

Shop around on the Internet. Always buy from a seller who a long time reputation for selling Lugol's Solution such as J.crow® or from an Iodoral seller who has a long relationship with the manufacturer, Optimox, so you get the true product, not a counterfeit.

Full disclosure: the charity I work for, Breast Cancer Choices, sells Iodoral as our charity fundraiser. Many people buy from us because as a nonprofit we can sell iodine cheaply, and the ten percent we make on sales goes to a good cause. I do not personally profit from any iodine product.

I've heard cabbage and the cruciferous vegetables cancel out iodine. Is that true?

As long as you're taking iodine, the goitrogenic (iodine blocking) vegetables will not suppress your thyroid or block iodine uptake. If you're not taking iodine, taking raw cruciferous vegetables or supplements made from these vegetables may block absorption of iodine to the thyroid. Unfortunately, some breast cancer patients have been known to take broccoli-based supplements without iodine, not understanding the consequences of blocking iodine.

What is Magnascent Iodine? Will it work as well as Lugol's or Iodoral?

Magnascent is a magnetized formulation that is usually used in addition to stronger forms of iodine/iodide. Magnascent was reportedly the formula used by Edgar Cayce. Some people report benefits from Magnascent, but if a person is seriously ill, no Iodine Literate Practitioner would recommend Magnascent as a standalone therapy.

Does decolorized (white iodine) work as well as Lugol's Iodine?

Decolorized iodine only contains potassium iodide. Lugol's and Iodoral contain both potassium iodide and elemental iodine. Patients with breast cysts have reported decolorized iodine does not work as well as Lugol's Iodine when used topically (on the skin).

I take thyroid medicine. Will iodine counteract that?

According to the iodine practitioners, no one has complained that iodine affects thyroid medication. The opposite has been reported. Iodine can be a missing link to make thyroid work better.

I spilled Lugol's Iodine on my kitchen counter. Is the stain permanent?

No. Usually making a thick paste of vitamin C powder and water will remove iodine stains. One of our Breast Cancer Think Tank members reports she removed a stain from her white bathroom rug by soaking the spot with Vitamin C paste, then letting it soak and sit.

What if a person has an auto immune thyroid disease such as Hashimoto's?

Originally, practitioners thought there might be a problem with Hashimoto's patients taking iodine. Now we've found that so-called problem is a myth perpetrated by those promoting an incomplete iodine protocol. After much study by the experienced iodine practitioners, it has become clear that iodine deficiency is often the most direct cause of Hashimoto's combined with selenium deficiency. Contact an Iodine Literate Practitioner who is experienced in using iodine for auto immune diseases. If your practitioner has not trained under the supervision of one of the major iodine doctors, he or she may not know the additional protocols for auto-immune disease, including the necessity of the right amount of selenium. Also, you may want to read this article with your doctor. *www.Optimox.com/pics/Iodine/IOD-22/ IOD_22.htm* or read Dr. Jeffrey Dach's easy to read explanation:

*/Jdach1.Typepad.com/natural_thyroid/2011/02/selenium-for-hashi
motos-thyroiditis-by-jeffrey-dach-md.html.* Many Hashi's patients
have also found eliminating gluten from the diet helps.

Do women need more iodine than men?
Boys and girls seem to require the same amount of iodine until
they reach puberty. As the breasts and ovaries begin to develop,
the iodine requirement goes up for the girls. The increased requirements can take iodine away from the thyroid at this time.
Goiter researcher, Dr. David Marine, found that Ohio girls and
boys experienced equal amounts of thyroid disease until the girls
reached puberty when significantly more girls developed goiter.
This discovery finally resulted in the iodization of salt in 1924.

Why do the breasts need iodine?
There are many iodine receptors in the breast to keep the milk
ducts and other tissue performing optimally. Iodine has been
observed to detoxify fluids in the breasts and eliminate cysts
which harbor toxins.

What does iodine deficiency have to do with the breast?
In animals, blocking dietary iodine will cause the breasts to
swell, develop nodules, fibrous tissue and cysts in a way that
parallels the progressive development of breast disease in
women. When iodine is supplied, the fibrocystic disease goes
away. When iodine is blocked again, the breast disease returns.

Do nursing women need more iodine?
In nursing mothers, the body will take iodine from the thyroid
if necessary in order to make sure the baby gets enough. It's one
reason some women hold onto post-baby weight. Less iodine
going to their thyroids and more to the baby via the breast could
slow down metabolism.

Iodine Stories

Meet, Lee: Her sleepiness, lumpy breasts, menstrual problems, thyroid disorder, depression ... all gone!

I'm a 47–year-old mother of four. I suffered for a couple decades with hypothyroidism and each time I went for my annual checkup, I would report the same: chronic sleepiness, brain fog, and increasing symptoms of estrogen dominance such as achy, lumpy breasts, and excessive menstrual bleeding. He would check my TSH only and send me on my way with a new anti-depressant and larger and larger amounts of Synthroid. I felt like what he gave me just wasn't helping and was never quite satisfied with his explanation of why he would not prescribe Armour or other glandular therapy.

I never went back and have been off all Synthroid for over a year. I went on the net to look for a new doctor but couldn't find one that took our insurance and would prescribe Armour. Then I found the Yahoo Iodine Group. The more I read, the more it became clear how I must be deficient in iodine, so I ordered some and started at the basic 12.5 mg dose of Iodoral.

After some mild detox symptoms, and starting the supplements and salt loading, I was feeling pretty good and decided to do the salt water detox protocol since I had many symptoms of bromide dominance. I have been on 50 mg for about a month. I am also taking over–the-counter thyroid glandular supplements. Let me say that I do not choose to be doing so on my own without a doctor's consult and approval, but I have found no other option.

The upside to my beginning the iodine protocol is that it has drastically changed my health for the better. I am now able to sweat for the first time. My basal temps are only a degree under normal now. My skin is much improved.

I am not bleeding as much during menstruation. Last time my period snuck up on me without any PMS or achy breasts. I am not craving sweets all the time and have lost 15 lbs. as I'm able to stick to a healthier diet. I would say the most profound change is the way my breasts have changed. They are smooth, soft, and not lumpy or achy anymore. I would describe it as "comfortable breasts." I can actually walk around without a bra and not hurt. I guess this is what it's like to feel "normal." I was probably on my way to breast cancer while I was in that condition.

I wanted to say "Thank You" to all of you at *BreastCancer Choices.org* for maintaining a site that discusses the detoxification protocol. I sure tried my best to find a doctor to help me get better, but, in lieu of that, I finally took charge of my own health. I will tell everyone I know to read the information about iodine. I know a lot of friends and relatives on Synthroid who are not even taking any iodine. If they are convinced, I will send them to your site.

You can share this testimonial with anyone you like and use my name also. Thanks again for saving my life!

Meet Ed: His "age-related hearing loss" drastically improves.

When I was 72, I was scheduled to be fitted with a hearing aid. A few days before my appointment, the hearing aid fitter called the house and needed to reschedule in five weeks because he was going into the hospital for an operation. Meanwhile, I had been taking 25 mg Iodoral and complained to my wife that I didn't notice anything. She said, so take another tablet. Before the hearing aid guy got back to work, my hearing loss disappeared so I cancelled the appointment and saved myself several thousand dollars.

Meet Gina from Norway: Many problems resolved from fibrocystic breasts to palpitations to candida.

I am not alone anymore! Thank you; I have learned a lot. I started on Iodine one year ago. Ailments: long time candida, Wilson's temperature syndrome, dry skin, FBD and so on. No doc involved; only my own research and experimental nature.

I started slow; didn't raise my dose to 50 mg until 6 months ago. Then the detox-thing kicked in; and more so when I upped my vitamin C from 1g to 6 to7g (bowel tolerance).

First noticeable changes after iodine:

Nails stopped splitting in layers, skin improved. Heart palpitations gone.

Temperature went up from average 36,5C to 37 C (98,7F)!!!
Allergy symptoms improved 70%(sneezing, sinus problems)

Fibrocystic breasts disease reduced by 90% when I raised to 50 mg.

Candida gone 90 %. I can live with the rest; it is under my control now!

Sun tolerance is 100% better; combined iodine and coconut oil is the best; no more burning for the sun-lover (I live in Norway and need it)

I also supplement with selenium, magnesium, pink salt, etc.
Other useful supplements:

Turmeric + enzymes; helps allergy symptoms, less sneezing + better digestion.

Borax; helps fungus related ailments/candida; combined with iodine.

Meet Don: Blood pressure, cholesterol and heart rate all normalized.

I have been using Lugol's, 240 mgs daily for about six months, my blood pressure and cholesterol have gotten into the normal range, my cholesterol was 220, now it is 180, my HDL has gone to 40, better than 35 before, my blood pressure was 150 over 90, I was on a low dosage of blood pressure meds to also slow my heart rate down, iodine seems to have fixed all three.

Meet Mary: 50 mg Iodine prevent genital herpes outbreaks, breast lumps, allergies, fatigue.

I'm excited to tell you that so long as I take 50 mg/day of Iodoral, I don't experience the genital herpes condition which has plagued me for many, many years. It hasn't been cured, but it's under control. I know this because I've only had herpes once since I started the Iodine Protocol nine months ago. That was when I tried after five months to reduce my dose to 37.5mg, I suffered a herpes breakout which resolved immediately when I brought my dosage back to 50mg of Iodoral.

Of course, this isn't the only benefit I've experienced since starting the Iodine Protocol, but it's probably the most exciting for me. I'm sure others will tell you of no more lumpy breasts and allergies and endless energy. I even give three drops of Lugol's 2% a day to my dogs!

Chapter Seven

FAQ 3
What Do Doctors Think
About Iodine?

What do most doctors think of iodine?

Most contemporary doctors were taught in medical school that iodine should be feared and could damage the thyroid. This fear (which Dr. Guy Abraham refers to as Iodophobia!) was the result of a policy change based on a study that proved mistaken and misleading. Fifty years ago, iodine was widely used for everything from ovarian cysts to hemorrhoids. Now the iodine information is getting exposure as patients report benefits back to their doctors.

My doctor says, "It's a fundamental law of physiology that iodine shuts down the thyroid."

That's what she was taught in medical school. Physiology is an ever-involving *theoretical* discipline of medicine. What your doctor learned about iodine as a fundamental, unquestioned law of physiology in medical school has turned out, (1) not to be fundamental, (2) not to be a law, and (3) completely refuted. Tens of thousands of iodine users have challenged the "law" by taking iodine in significant milligram dosages to great benefit.

Be patient with your doctor. It takes years for the medical profession to catch up with new information. You may remember how long it took for Doctors Barry Marshall and Robin Warren to convince the medical profession that peptic ulcers were caused not from psychological causes but by a specific bacterium. They finally received the Nobel Prize in 2005. A lot of us are hoping Dr. Guy Abraham will be recognized in the same way.

I wanted to try iodine but my doctor said it was just an Internet fad.

Does he mean that the thousands of people have discovered something that made them feel better should be disregarded because they discovered it on the internet? If iodine supplementation were a fad, it wouldn't have been used continuously from the 1820s to the 1940s.

Why doesn't my doctor know about iodine?

1. Because he or she has not attended Integrative Medicine conferences.
2. Because iodine is so cheap, can't be patented, requires no prescription and thus no drug company sales rep has come to the doctor's office pushing it.
3. Because he or she still believes the debunked Wolff-Chaikoff conclusion, claiming iodine will damage the thyroid, is accurate.

But Iodine literacy is spreading fast. At the November 2010 ACAM (American College for the Advancement of Medicine) conference, integrative medicine expert, Michael Schachter, MD, asked the audience doctors how many of them used iodine in their practices. Half of the audience members raised their hands. Great progress!

Has the information about iodine been presented at any medical conferences?

Yes. To name a few: The ACAM Conferences, The Anti-Aging Conferences, The Weston. A. Price Conference, The Iodine Conferences and others.

Are there are any medical studies I can show my doctor?

It would depend on what your goals as a patient are. You may have to research your particular concern and bring it to the attention of the patient-to-patient experts in the online iodine community.

Where can I find an Iodine Literate Practitioner?

Look in Part 4, the *Resources* section of this book or go to *www.Breast CancerChoices.org/IPractitioners* where the list is constantly updated.

Iodine Stories

Meet Katy: Tumor size reduced.

My doctor in 2008 wanted me to take Tamoxifen to reduce the size of my breast tumor before surgery. I was very resistant to taking the Tamoxifen. Finally, I bought the prescription and took it home. My husband really wanted me to do what the doctor said. So I did try the Tamoxifen for about a week. It caused a toxic problem for me. It created what is known as Tamoxifen-induced asthma.

I was staying at a quaint and peaceful mountain cabin at the time. We were doing day hikes. I scared the bejesus out of my husband when I began having trouble breathing on one of our hikes. He and I thought I was going to die right then and there. I had no idea that Tamoxifen could cause something like that.

But by Googling Tamoxifen and asthma, I found that research was done that identified Tamoxifen induced asthma as a serious side effect. The next day I was on the phone with the doctor. Her solution was to take half a dose. I decided to screw that and after just a week on Tamoxifen, I went off of it ... period. No more asthma ... period.

In the meantime, I had been taking Lugol's iodine at higher and higher doses by mouth as well as painting it on my breast. After three to four months when I went back to the doctor, my tumor had indeed reduced from 2.7 cm down to 0.8 cm. You could clearly feel the difference in size too. The doctor, however, came unglued when I told her I had not taken the Tamoxifen and also that I would not take it. She yelled at me that I would be begging her for Tamoxifen when I had metastases all over my body and was in great pain, etc., etc. It was a frightening nightmare that even after three years I get all stressed out even thinking about it. The doctor said she would schedule the surgery, and I wondered why I should have surgery at this point. Why wouldn't I continue to work at shrinking the tumor to nothing?

This was the icing on the cake. She told me that no one can do that. That anyone who tried alternative means always ended up having to come back to her to have it cut out! Yikes! Finally, she said that she would give me eight weeks to shrink the tumor then she would cut it out. Ha! I have yet to have surgery. And I am alive and well. I could tell you more of the story. But the meadow is calling.

Please just start taking your iodine now. Don't wait!

Meet Connie: Uterine fibroids resolved along with endometrial lining normalizing.

I got rid of my uterine fibroids plus my endometrial lining thinned out and was now normal. It took about six months.

Meet Raymond. His goiter shrank 90 percent. Hemorrhoids are gone.

I am by no means an expert, but what I can say is that HIGH dose iodine shrank my thyroid goiter by 90 percent, and my hemorrhoids are gone, so, it's been working pretty darn well for me!

I take about 130 mg a day and the companion nutrients, especially the unrefined sea salt. I split my dose between Iodoral and Lugol's. I figure if I do it that way, I have a better chance of killing nasties in the stomach. If you just take the Iodoral, it passes the stomach and goes directly to the small intestine. So, I get a one-two punch.

I will not always take this much, but right now I'm trying to kill pathogens, shrink tumors, and push out bromine and other toxic halides. I had a lot of detox symptoms ... acne, rash, sinus pain and pressure, aches and pains BUT I pushed through to the other side and I'm doing much better now. I used salt flushes to lessen the discomfort. The first week, my thyroid goiter swelled up and it hurt. I got scared. I almost stopped BUT I knew that SOMETHING was happening with my thyroid which had to mean it was using the iodine in some way, so I gave it time and then suddenly it profoundly shrank. Other people have also experienced the shrinking of goiters very quickly.

Meet Carla: Her ovarian cysts and fibrocystic breast condition ... now undetectable.

After my hysterectomy in 1987, the doctor told me that I had ovarian cysts. Since then, at my last exam, the doctor said there weren't any there. They could be felt before. I also do not have the stabbing pains I had in the past.

In regards to fibrocystic breast tissue, a doctor told me during an exam that I had, she felt them. Again, at last exam the doctor said there was no sign of it. All pain and lumps are gone.

Chapter Eight

FAQ 4
How Do People
Supplement Iodine?

How much Iodine do most iodine takers use to start?

Most veteran iodine users would say start with a low dose such as 12.5 mg and build up. Others start at 50 mg and feel fine. Others take even more to feel their best. Many doctors recommend starting with the salt loading protocol for two weeks before beginning iodine.

What is the Iodine Protocol?

The Iodine Protocol is the guideline for iodine takers presented by the principal iodine doctors at the 2007 Iodine Conferences. The protocol covers the amounts of iodine and companion nutrients the experienced iodine prescribers found effective. This protocol has withstood the test of time with most patients and Iodine Literate Practitioners.

Is there a test for iodine deficiency?

The most reliable test is the 24 hour Iodine Loading Test. This test is sometimes used in conjunction with other tests. The iodine loading test must be evaluated by an Iodine Literate Practitioner and repeated after a course of iodine supplementation. At Breast Cancer Choices, we occasionally see people whose first test isn't so bad, but when they test a few months later after supplementation, the iodine saturation number drops lower discouraging them. But it appears that the first test was misleading because the iodine absorption tissues were so damaged or atrophied that the much of the test dosage of Iodoral passed through the body unabsorbed into the urine.

Damaged NIS symporter tissues may be compared to an old, dry sponge. Water runs right off it until it is moist.

An experienced Iodine Literate Practitioner will be able to explain why the loading test results may move from high to low, then back up to high again. The goal is to make sure absorption trends upward after the second test. The Iodine Doctors find the companion nutrients speed up the process.

Takeaway info on the Iodine Loading Test: be sure your practitioner knows about the need for periodic retesting until your levels are in the normal range.

How does the average person begin taking iodine?
See the following example:

Kathy started taking Iodine under the direction of an Iodine Literate Practitioner. She began by drinking a quarter teaspoon of salt dissolved in eight ounces of water twice a day for fourteen days before starting with Optimox brand Iodoral tablets. He suggested the Iodoral because it is the most predictable formulation for starting iodine dosing.

Her doctor instructed her to start with one 12.5 mg tablet and take it for two weeks along with the salt water. She was also instructed to take the iodine companion nutrients:

300-600 Mg magnesium
1 tab Optimox ATP Cofactors twice a day
200 mcg selenium (or selenomethionine)
1,000 mg Vitamin C 3 times per day
½ teaspoon of salt per day with food
Additional ¼ teaspoon of salt twice per day
in eight oz. water.

After two weeks, he asked her if she felt any reactions. She didn't, so he raised the dosage to two 12.5 mg tablets for a total of 25 mg. After another two weeks, she was instructed to raise the dose again and only report back if she had side effects. If she didn't, she was instructed to raise the Iodoral to four tablets for a total of 50 mg.

At this point, Kathy began to get brain fog and a headache. Her doctor told her she could take the salt water twice a day but stop taking all Iodoral on weekends to flush out toxins the iodine may have dislodged. Breast Cancer Choices' "pulse-dosing strategy" caused all side effects to go away.

She is now able to take 50 mg Iodoral every day but she skips one weekend every once in a while as per her doctor's instructions.

Should I take iodine with food?

Most people take iodine with food. However, if you are taking Iodoral which was designed to be easy on the stomach, you may have no problem on an empty stomach.

What time of the day should I take iodine?

Iodine is usually taken in the morning. Some people have reported that taking iodine later in the day has kept them awake at night.

Why did Lugol's Iodine Solution mixed in water upset my stomach?

Stomach distress has been reported many times with Lugol's. That's why the coated Iodoral tablet was invented. Sometimes just taking Lugol's on a full stomach may help. You may find other brands of iodine which have a similar coating. If any product is irritating your stomach, the manufacturers advise you to **discontinue taking it immediately.**

Can I take iodine any other way than by mouth?

Iodine is often applied to the skin. Some iodine gets in the bloodstream this way. Topical application is often used by people who are hesitant to take iodine by mouth or want to slow down the absorption of iodine. Much iodine is lost by evaporation this way but it has shown to be surprisingly effective in an emergency.

Historically, iodine has also been compounded into rectal or vaginal suppositories for local use.

When using iodine products such as Lugol's Solution on the skin, the experts recommend mixing it with a small amount of oil in the palm of your hand first, then applying it. This method is reported to reduce the chance of irritation. Grapeseed oil, castor oil, jojoba oil or coconut oil make good "carriers" for Lugol's Solution.

When can I stop taking iodine supplements?
The usual advice is to only take iodine supplements for as long as you want to be healthy (a healthcare professional's attempt at humor in an otherwise serious subject).

Can my pet take iodine? How much?
Dr. David Brownstein reports that pets have been given Lugol's Iodine at a dosage of 0.08 mg /per pound. Several reports have come in about chickens and parrots preferring Lugol's treated water. Livestock owners may be familiar with how iodine enhances animal health and reproduction capacities. The veterinary use of iodine goes back decades.

Should I take tyrosine with iodine?
Some practitioners suggest taking tyrosine, but others suggest avoiding tyrosine if you have any concerns about breast cancer or melanoma. These cancers are in the same biologic family, and melanoma can be very difficult to treat. Concerns exist that tyrosine can aggravate any melanoma.

What are these "Iodine Symporters" I read about on the Internet?
According to iodine experts, the symporters are the tissues used by the body to trap iodine from the bloodstream so it can be absorbed by the body. Unfortunately, over time, these tissues can become damaged by pollutants (think rust) or become scarce, causing the body to become iodine deficient. In order to heal, the iodine absorbing tissues, supplementing iodine is necessary in combination with antioxidants.

Competition for the receptors that absorb iodine is fierce. The halogen group of elements is controlled by a mechanism called "competitive inhibition." Bromine usually wins this competition because of its prevalence as an environmental toxin. But chlorine, fluorine and the lesser known astatine can knock iodine off this very appealing receptor.

As long as bromine dominates the receptors, iodine deficiency prevails, so the goal is to overpower and displace the bromine so iodine can get absorbed.

My first Iodine Loading Test came back at 75 percent saturation. Then after three months taking Iodine, I took another Loading Test and the saturation dropped to 50 percent. How can I have less iodine in my body?

We think the initial test may reflect iodine deficiency symporter atrophy which resolves as iodine repairs the absorption tissues.

In our Iodine Investigation Project, we have collected a lot of data on breast cancer patients taking iodine. Occasionally, the loading test after three months reports the iodine level dropped from the first test. A 75 percent saturation might drop to a 50 percent saturation on the second test. Then the third test result will show an increase.

At the Iodine Conference, one of the doctors mentioned this happened to his own loading tests and some of his patients. What this seems to mean is that the tissues which absorb iodine aren't working. So the iodine just washes right past the absorbers and shows up in the urine, showing a false lab value. Think of water flowing over a dry sponge, not absorbing until it gets more water. The iodine absorbing tissues may atrophy until they get nourished.

Once iodine and antioxidants start repairing the absorbing tissues, the Iodine Loading Tests will show how much iodine is being absorbed. That will be a more accurate reading of iodine saturation.

If a patient is clearly iodine deficient, some practitioners will not even begin to test patients' iodine levels for three months.

Is there a test that can measure whether I'm absorbing iodine efficiently?

A new testing concept has been developed called the saliva/serum iodide ratio test. Both 24 hour urine finds are compared with blood iodide levels and saliva iodide levels. Ask your doctor if you are a candidate for this test. This link explains the test: *www.Optimox.com/pics/Iodine/IOD-13/IOD_13.htm*

Can I apply iodine topically to my breasts?

Applying Lugol's Solution directly to the breast with a brush has been used for at least 150 years for breast pain. In a pinch, when Lugol's Solution is unavailable, some women have applied Tincture of Iodine. Many report it helps to mix the iodine in your palm with an oil such as jojoba or grapeseed oil to help prevent possible irritation. Tip: iodine can stain. Don't wear your favorite bra while using iodine topically. Lugol's stains can usually be removed by applying a paste of vitamin C powder.

What is the Funahashi Method? (The Lugol's–Progesterone Method)

"The Funahashi Method" is an invention of the Grass Roots Iodine Movement used to rapidly speed up the shrinking of breast cysts. It should be more accurately called the Lugol's-Progesterone Method. Dr. Funahashi has absolutely no connection to the method named for his experiments which were proven to have subsequently been shown in patient-to-patient communication to benefit women.

Dr. H. Funahashi found progesterone enhanced the uptake of iodine to tumors in animals which subsequently shrank. The Lugol's-Progesteone Method should be undertaken under the supervision of an Iodine Literate Practitioner who has an understanding of bioidentical hormones.

The Lugol's-Progesterone Method involves applying a small amount of progesterone to the breasts along with the topical application of Lugol's Iodine until the cyst disappears. 50 mg of Lugol's or Iodoral by mouth are used along with topical applications. The uptake of iodine by progesterone has been observed in other hormone dependent tissues such as the ovaries and uterus. (See Brown-Grant and Rogers, 1972).

What about the Prostate?

Iodine has been used for over 100 years for prostate disease. Recent reports of Lugol's Iodine and Iodoral reducing the symptoms of benign prostate disease (BPH) have been coming more frequent. When one five-year iodine taker, an eighty-year-old man, told his doctor he only got up once a night to urinate, she did not believe him and said he must have forgotten, "because no 80 year-old man gets up only once."

Can local application help there also?

A number of men have found an increased effect using Lugol's Iodine topically to the testicles with a carrier oil to avoid irritation.

What is the T2T Method? (testicle-to-testicle method) is a method of iodine application to the skin named for online iodine activist, T2T. He experimented with applying 20 drops Lugol's Iodine to one testicle one night, the other testicle the next night, alternating in order to enhance sexual performance. The T2T method has been modified by another activist, "G," to add grapeseed oil to the formulation to prevent irritation and increase absorption. Other men have tried this and reported good results. However, with all health strategies, consult your medical professional.

What more can I read?

Please go to the *Resources* section of this book (Part 4) and read *The Iodine Loading Test.*

Are there side effects of iodine supplementation?

Like any nutrient, sometimes people experience side effects. It's important to understand most symptoms are due to the iodine detoxing the bromine and toxins faster than the kidneys and liver can handle it. The Salt Loading Protocol usually addresses detoxification issues.

Please see the *side effects* section in *Resources*, Part 4, for the Iodine Related Bromide Detox.

What are the companion nutrients and do I absolutely need them?

The companion nutrients include specific amounts of Vitamin C, niacin, riboflavin, and magnesium along with the Salt Loading Protocol. Patients report these specific nutrients boost iodine absorption. See the *Resources* pages for specific dosages.

What is the difference between consuming refined salt and taking unrefined salt in the salt loading protocol?

The Iodine Literate Practitioners recommend using only un-processed, unbleached, unrefined salt, free of anti-caking and bleaching agents. It is sometimes called Celtic Salt or sea salt. Redmond's Real Salt is a brand many people like. But many "gourmet," unprocessed, unrefined salts are available through-out all over the world. Supplementing unrefined salt is part of the companion nutrient strategy and different from the salt loading protocol. The supplementary salt appears to support the adrenals. Many unrefined salt-taking patients report feeling better, perhaps due to the many minerals in unrefined salt that are not found in commercial, processed salt.

Why did my doctor prescribe iodine tablets and never mention taking salt water or the companion nutrients?

A lot of practitioners don't understand the Iodine Protocol. They may not even know there is a protocol when prescribing iodine and have not read the Iodine Project Papers, the Iodine Protocol or Dr. Brownstein's *Iodine* book and never consult the online user groups. A couple of weeks on any of the user groups would provide good training in why taking iodine is not always as easy as taking a single pill. **The biggest problem the iodine-taking community faces is the common belief that there is nothing to know about iodine.**

I have high blood pressure and have restricted salt. The salt loading scares me. Help?

If unprocessed salt is taken **in proportion** to the right amount of water, you should not have any problem. The water acts somewhat like a diuretic. Be sure to consult your iodine-literate practitioner. Read *Salt Your Way to Health* by David Brownstein, MD.

Do I have to keep taking iodine for life?

As far as we know, you need to take iodine for as long as it takes to build up and maintain tissue stores. Given our constant exposure to bromines, this will probably be a long time. Some people have been able to reduce their dosages after a few years when their Iodine Loading tests shows 90 percent saturation. The general rule is take iodine only as long as you want to be healthy and protect yourself against the daily bombardment of toxins (such as bromines) which disrupt body functions. The importance of avoiding bromine exposure is discussed later in the book.

What is the most important thing to know about taking iodine?

You should know what is going on in your body when you supplement iodine. If you know what the process and strategy is, you will be ready for it and know how to handle it.

The answer to that question varies with the individual. But from corresponding with thousands of iodine takers, the salt-loading protocol (taking a certain amount of salt water periodically) has been the most helpful in relieving and detoxing symptoms of bromide and other impurities which iodine pushes from the cells.

In my family, I've seen salted water get rid of brain fog or a headache within a half hour.

The salt water method has been used for over a hundred years. Most recently the US Army used an intravenous sodium solution when the Gulf War soldiers got bromide toxicity from Pyrodostigmine bromium medication prescribed to protect against a possible nerve gas attack. See "A Review of the Scientific Literature As It Pertains to Gulf War Illnesses" by Beatrice Golomb, MD, PhD.

I can't repeat this enough: at Breast Cancer Choices' Iodine Investigation Project, we developed the "pulse-dosing" technique to remedy detox symptoms. Pulse dosing means stopping iodine (but not the salt loading protocol or companion nutrients) for 48 hours to flush toxins from the kidneys.

Do I still need iodine if I take thyroid medication?

Some believe thyroid medication makes the body metabolize iodine faster so it's even more important to take iodine if you are currently taking thyroid medication.

Which parts of the body does iodine affect?

Iodine inhabits every cell of the body. Some organs require more iodine than others but it's hard to say which part of any individual's body may need more, as some people may show, for example, obvious deficiencies in the breast, and in others it will show up in the skin or other organs.

More Iodine Stories

Meet Sue: Energy returns, breasts soften, dermoid cyst disappears.

I'm a 45 year-old female. I heard about iodine on the net and thought it probably can't hurt since so many others on the Cure-zone Iodine Forum web site had been using it for years. I tried iodine to see if it would work on my lumpy breasts. When I first took 50 mg Iodoral, I got a huge surge of mental energy. Not like caffeine, just clear thinking. I didn't realize I had been that slow-brained before. I'm a writer so this brain boost really came in handy. It took about three months before my breasts became squishy again. This is a relief because I was nervous that inflamed breasts might lead to cancer. My skin also got clearer and a dermoid cyst I've had on my waist suddenly wasn't there.

Meet Mindy: Graves' Disease symptoms improve.

I was diagnosed with Graves' Disease about a year ago and a few months after that, my right eye became swollen and exhibited mild exophthalmos. I recently began taking 25 mg Iodoral with Vitamin C, magnesium, selenium and sea salt. I've noticed that my pulse has slowed down from 88 to 78 and that I don't need 9 hours of sleep anymore.

Meet Frank: Prostatitus improves. Less nighttime urination. Hair regrowth.

I have not posted this anywhere yet. Iodine cured my prostate problems, called prostatitus. My symptoms were weak urine flow, starting & stopping, three or more trips to the bathroom every night. I slowly titrated iodine from ½ mg to 50 mg over a four month period, going slow to prevent detox symptoms. After 3 months and iodine at 25 mg daily with required supplements, it was clear that my prostate problems were fading away.

After 4 months of iodine at 50mg daily, my prostate problems are GONE. Now I only get up once in the night, and even last all night without getting up at times. Urine flow is great, and life is good!

Also, my hair seems to be growing in.

Meet Charlene: Hypothyroid disease with autoimmune antibodies resolves, breast scan goes from a high risk level 4 to level 1.

I wanted to tell you my success story, to encourage you to keep getting the news out about Iodorol. I am hypothyroid and have been seeing a holistic MD for the past 3 years. He put me on Iodorol (I take 50 mg/day) for my thyroid antibodies, breast health, and because I live in Michigan (the Goiter Belt).

Two years ago I got my first thermoscan (infrared mammography) that was a Level 4 on one side. It scared me half to death!

My MD increased my iodine, had me take Calcium d-glucarate, and 6 months of Oncoplex. I am happy to report after 6 months my thermoscan down-graded to level 3, and now a year and a half later, it is a level one—normal on both sides! Not only that, the thyroid antibodies are no longer showing up in my blood work. I am thanking the Lord, and being faithful with my Iodorol & ATP co-factors, which I've also been taking for a few years.

Thought you would like a success story!

Meet Mary Ann: Extreme bladder issues and pain, fertility issues, low basal temperature, history of irregular periods, fibrocystic breasts, ovarian cysts, mood and energy issues. Now on the mend.

I believe that my misadventures with iodine deficiency began with early (just turned 10) menses—very painful and heavy. The next few years I had irregular periods—no periods for months at a time—ovarian cysts—was underweight, had low basal temp, low blood pressure, low blood sugar, and slow heart rate.

Had trouble conceiving until I finally got my weight up to 105 (age 24, 5' 4", medium frame). Had typical thyroid issues that follow pregnancies and breast feeding.

Had my first bladder infection at age 18—and have been in a living nightmare of recurrent infections, misdiagnoses, bladder neck polyps, extreme and painful treatments, WAY too many anti-biotics, and enough pain at times to make me consider suicide.

NOW I discover that bladder issues like mine are also a symptom of iodine deficiency—and that iodine therapy not only reverses the cause but treats the bladder and infections—including urethral and bladder spasms. I can only imagine, but I think these spasms may be similar to prostate issues.

I have had my urethra spasm so hard that it clamped down and shut off urine flow. I have had to high tail it to the ER for an immediate catheterization—or literally face a ruptured bladder.

As you might imagine, the cath bag would look more like blood than urine.

So NOW I find that the answer all along has been iodine. And, even just ten days into 12.5 mg iodine/iodide therapy, I feel more comfortable with my bladder/urethra that I can remember feeling in years. Better mood and energy too.

Meet Monica: Suffering from Paget's Disease, a kind of breast cancer affecting the skin, it improved in three months. See Figure 3.

Back in 2009 my endocrinologist decided to lower my thyroid meds because of the TSH test (I am thyroidless) and consequently destroyed my entire endocrine system in the process. It was about the time I first reported my flakey nipple to the doctor that does my mammograms and whole breast ultrasound.

Fast forward to 2012, I decided I was tired of the flakey nipple that I assumed was eczema and went to see a dermatologist. She prescribed several different types of creams over a few months. The symptoms would disappear momentarily then return. It was finally decided to do a biopsy. On July 5th, 2012, the verdict was in. I was diagnosed with Paget's disease.

Per the lab report: The S-100 stain demonstrates epidermal and dermal Langerhans cells. The Cytokeratin stain is positive. Cytokeratin-7 stain is focally positive. The Estrogen receptor stain also focally positive. The Progesterone receptor stain is focally weakly positive. The Gross Cystic Disease fluid protein stain is negative. The Mart-1 stain is negative. The CEA stain is strongly positive. The results were confirmed by a second lab two weeks later.

I was sent for an MRI immediately. Nothing has ever shown up on the mammogram or ultrasound. The MRI showed asymmetric flattening of the nipple with periareolar edema and contrast enhancement compatible with given diagnosis of Paget's disease. Retroarolar intraductal carcinoma is not seen. A round 1.1 x 0.8 cm right level one axillary lymph node is suspicious. There are scattered cysts, approximately 15. There is abnormal skin thickening and enhancement seen in the right Breast anteriorly over an area of approximately 6 cm x 4 cm in transverse and AP dimensions respectively.

There is, however, no significant non-masslike enhancement in the retroarolar right breast to suggest extensive ductal carcinoma in situ.

When I received my diagnosis, I was immediately sent to the surgeon. The course of action was either partial removal of the breast with reconstruction to include radiation or the other option, a mastectomy.

The doctor who does my mammograms wanted me to have a bi-lateral mastectomy because I take natural hormones supplements. The oncologist had the same opinion about removing my breast. I also had two other doctors telling me to remove my breast, before I decided I was probably doing this alone.

I do not do anything these days without researching the alternatives after what was done to me in 2009. It has been a long road back to health. I know from my compromised immune system that I am still working on, radiation was not for me.

I have been under the guidance of a remarkable nutritionist and a naturopathic doctor since 2009. I had been taking iodine, but only 225 mcg. About a month after my diagnosis, I started taking 37.5 mg of Iodoral and then 2 weeks later upped it to 50 mg of Iodoral where I remain today. Approximately a month after my diagnosis, I started painting my breasts with Lugol's Solution at the direction of my nutritionist.

I was putting it straight on with a Q-tip to start out. Later, I learned about carrier oils and now apply it after I butter up with coconut oil. My iodine loading test showed full saturation in September.

The changes to my breast were amazing. At first, the area looked horrible. I had large patches of dark dead skin that eventually sloughed off. Within a few months, my breast looked pretty much normal, with the exception that my nipple is not the normal dark color. My hopes are that with continued use of the Iodine with changes in diet and detoxing, that I can get this under manageable control. Only time will tell. Right now I am feeling pretty good.

Figure 3
Monica's Paget's Disease before Iodine therapy, August 2012, and after, October 2012.

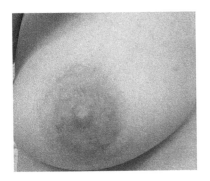 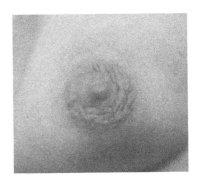

Chapter Nine

FAQ 5
What Happens When
You Take Iodine?

1. **Remember that competitive situation between Iodine and Bromine?** When iodine supplementation builds up in your bloodstream, iodine will "chase" bromine off its seats on the receptors. As they compete for the same seats, iodine chases bromine into the bloodstream. Bromine goes on the run in your body like an escaped rat, looking for a new place to sit. If displaced bromine isn't excreted through the kidneys fast enough, it will seat itself in the bloodstream, thyroid, brain, skin, etc., and you may get symptoms.

2. **Die-Off Detox:** Iodine also possesses antibiotic, antiparisitic, antifungal and antiviral properties and can displace metals. So several detoxification actions can occur at the same time as bromide is escaping your tissues as iodine chases it.

3. **Bromide Sedation:** Bromide is also sedating and was used in the early 1900s as a sedative, so if you absorb the detoxified bromine faster than you excrete it, symptoms such as headaches, fatigue or runny nose can occur. Brain

fog or sedation may be a result of the bromine that was sequestered quietly in your tissues suddenly getting mobilized into your bloodstream and making you feel dopey. A more complete list of iodine-related detoxification symptoms can be found in Part 4, *Resources*.

4. **Mood changes** have been reported by some. As always, when the symptoms get uncomfortable, the iodine patient activists have found stopping iodine and using the Salt Loading Protocol to be an effective remedy.

Sometimes (not always) bromides and other toxins get "stuck." When detoxed bromides, dead microbes and metals can't get out of your body fast enough, they appear to get *trapped* on the way out of your body. This is when symptoms occur and detox needs to be intensified to release the trapped bromides into your body's detoxification pathways such as the kidneys and liver. Salt water and Vitamin C have been shown to help excrete bromides. Others report that 500 mg niacin or the ATP Cofactors help. Zinc has proved helpful for skin problems. Both the Curezone Iodine Forum and The Yahoo Iodine Group have found that detox pathways such as the liver should be cleaned up. See the iodine online groups for other detox strategies such as saunas, detox formulas and herbs.

Remember, detoxification is a good thing. Getting rid of toxins makes the organs stronger and enhances the absorption of iodine and other nutrients. Again, not everyone experiences detoxification symptoms.

Read more about Iodine Related Bromide and Toxin Detoxification Symptoms in the *Resources* section of this book.

More Iodine Stories

Meet Jim: Increased testosterone levels.

There is no question iodine increases testosterone. I've raised my free and total Testosterone 60 percent since starting iodine 12 months ago (monthly blood work). Still have a ways to go to get into range for my age. I'm now taking 100 mg of iodine.

There is no doubt iodine has been the most important component. I took a very conservative approach initially and started with single mg level dosages, but only experienced noticeable changes when getting to 50 to 100 mg levels. Scale up as quickly as possible while keeping detox manageable.

I take tribulus, fenugreek, damiana, American ginseng and maca along with the iodine.

Meet Howard: Heart rhythm disorder (atrial fibrillation) improves.

I've had atrial fib for about 20 years after several bouts with Lyme Disease. After a few months of taking 50 mg Iodoral, my doctor listened and said, "Your heart beat seems fairly even today. Are you doing anything different?" I said taking iodine and he brushed it off.

The next time I visited he remarked that my heart was much more even again. I repeated that the only thing I'm doing different is taking Iodoral. He said he would investigate the relationship between iodine and afib. He took about a year to research. Now he prescribes iodine regularly to many of his patients for many different complaints. Author's note: many studies exist associating iodine deficiency with cardiovascular disease. For a review, see Cann, SA, (2006).

Meet Grace: Wrist pain improves.

I already had a C5-6 fusion surgery 10 years ago. Things were getting worse again. The pain was getting so bad and the numbness was going more up my arm, into my elbow. However, after putting the iodine/coconut oil on my wrist, I don't know, I may just not even need the MRI the doctor is contemplating.

Now, maybe I won't even need anything more than the iodine! I also put some more on this morning, and now it feels great. When at the computer and using the mouse, it causes a lot of strain on my right forearm, too. Hopefully, that won't hurt so much anymore, either.

I also decided that since it helped my arm that I would put some on my neck, near where they did the fusion surgery. Fatigue is the reason I originally decided to add the Iodine Protocol to the Low Dose Naltrexone because it had helped so much, and others who took it had been helped by the iodine.

Meet John: Allergies disappearing, cherry angiomas falling off.

I have remained off of all allergy medications—using only oral iodine, Ponaris iodized emollient nasal oil, and iodized Miracell ear care oil since this past Monday. My allergy symptoms continue to improve daily—and I need less Ponaris each day—even while the spring pollen count goes up.

Even though the count is still low/medium, in the past, I would have already started to get more symptomatic. The pollen forecast here indicates that next week the pollen count will be very high, which will tell me even more about my allergy status. I am NOT staying indoors with the windows shut and the air system clearing the air. I have the windows open and am spending time outdoors. I probably will close the house and clean the air when the pollen count goes above medium.

I mentioned before that I have a few small and a very few, bigger—cherry angiomas—have had them since my mid 40s. Some of the smallest ones are drying up and flaking off now when I shower with a wash cloth. So, I have started treating a few of the larger ones with tincture of iodine to see what happens to them. Also, in Dr. Brownstein's *Salt* book, he recommends sea salt & hydrogen peroxide in bathwater to detox through the skin. I'm going to try that, too.

Meet Jesse: Hair loss stopped. Body temperature normalizes.

The main benefit I have noticed so far is cessation of hair loss when I wash my hair. My temp has risen to almost normal. I have excess fat on my tummy which was cold to touch. A Chinese medicine practitioner told me this should be warm, but I was unsuccessful in warming it up until I started the iodine. Now it is toasty warm to touch. I am hoping this means it might disappear in due course!

Meet Belinda: Painful breasts, hypothyroidism, 50 pounds excess weight resolved.

Thank you for introducing me to iodine. At 54, my breasts were like balls of rocks and I was 50 pounds overweight. I was diagnosed as hypothyroid but the medication never did anything. Then I was diagnosed with breast cancer. I began taking Iodoral because it was the main part of my integrative doctor's supplement protocol.

I experienced a little brain fog detox when I started because I skipped the salt water part of the iodine protocol. Then I started it and all the brain fog went away. Gradually, my weight just came down to normal. I was so thrilled that when I had an all-women birthday party, I bought little bottles of Iodoral as party favors. I'm one of those people who tells strangers about iodine because it changed my life.

Chapter Ten

FAQ 6
What Are the Side Effects
of Taking Iodine?

How do people get rid of any side effects that
occur while first taking iodine?

1. **"Salt Loading"** The use of the **salt loading method**
   to escort bromide out of the body fast has been used
   for over a hundred years. When Gulf War soldiers
   experienced bromide toxicity from the experimental
   use of Pyridostigmine Bromide (supposedly a nerve
   gas protectant) the Army used a salt solution IV as a
   detox agent.

   Salt water "captures" the bromide so it doesn't
   lodge back in the system. If you take the salt loading
   protocol, you should prevent most, if not all, of the
   bromide detox effect. Some doctors even recommend
   using the salt loading procedure before starting iodine
   supplementation. See the Salt Loading recipe in Part 4,
   the *Resources* section of this book.

2. **Reduce the iodine dosage and build up gradually.**

3. **Pulse-dose** That means try taking no iodine for 48 hours to flush the kidneys and other detoxification pathways—then restarting. Many iodine users have found this tip very effective. Some report feeling a kind of euphoria after the 48 hour iodine detox/rest period.

What is unrefined salt?

Any salt that has unprocessed or unrefined marked on the label. Redmond's Real Salt or Celtic Salt are two well known brands. Trader Joe's also sells a nice coarse, unrefined sea salt from France. Please read *Salt Your Way to Health*, by David Brownstein, MD, available at *www.DrBrownstein.com* for an exciting read on why salt is a powerful and misunderstood vital nutrient.

Do I need to take ½ teaspoon unrefined salt on the iodine protocol even if I'm taking the salt loading protocol?

The extra unrefined salt is highly recommended by the iodine doctors and the Yahoo Iodine Group. The extra salt supports the adrenals and helps the rest of the nutrients work better.

What do I do if I get side effects from iodine supplementation?

Make sure you have an Iodine Literate Practitioner who knows how to use salt water and the iodine companion nutrients in conjunction with iodine supplementation. Make sure he understands that "pulse dosing" (stopping iodine for 48 hours) is often effective for detox symptoms. See the Salt Loading Protocol in Part 4, the *Resources* section of this book.

I felt sluggish while taking more than 12.5 mg iodine? What's going on?

If you understand how iodine supplementation works, you will be better prepared to manage any possible detox symptoms with your doctor. Review the *Salt Loading Protocol* in the *Resources* section, Part 4. Often using the salt water recipe (salt loading protocol) combined with a two day stop from iodine will banish any sluggishness or brain fog. Thousands of iodine takers report this result.

I started taking iodine for breast cysts two weeks ago and my breasts are becoming more tender. Shouldn't my breasts be feeling the opposite?

A small but measurable number of participants of Breast Cancer Choices' Iodine Investigation Project have reported temporary breast tenderness. I'm not aware of any iodine takers whose breast pain continued after taking iodine for several months if they took iodine along with the recommended companion nutrients. I'm sure there must be some women whose breasts don't respond to iodine. I just haven't heard from them.

We think that some iodine deficient breasts accustomed to iodine scarcity expand temporarily to trap as much iodine as possible. We've called this a "post scarcity effect." Once the breasts get accustomed to a sufficient iodine supply the swelling resolves. This is only a working theory on the basis of how the body adapts to other types of nutrient or calorie restriction as an adaptation and survival mechanism.

After a week of supplementing iodine, I got an odd swallowing sensation. What is that?

This effect has been reported in a percentage of patients. It isn't clear if the swelling is a bromide detox effect as the tissues get re-organized, or if it is the "post scarcity effect" of the thyroid trying to trap as much iodine as possible, as fast as possible, in an attempt to compensate for any future iodine "famines." Again, once the thyroid learns it will be getting a steady supply of iodine, the swelling goes down. Check with your Iodine Literate Practitioner.

After taking iodine, the ferritin level on my blood test dropped. Why?

Ferritin levels dropping have been reported several times. While the exact reason is unknown, the belief is that the metabolic boost that iodine restores may make the body use more than its usual amount of iron. The Yahoo Iodine Group recommends taking a B complex vitamin plus Floradix Iron plus Herbs along with food until ferritin levels stabilize.

I took iodine for my breasts, and my family doctor said my TSH blood test showed it made me hypothyroid.

Elevated TSH blood tests have been reported numerous times in people supplementing with iodine. This doesn't necessarily mean you are going hypo. TSH changes can mean your body is changing as it accommodates this abundance of a precious nutrient. Usually the reference range for free T3 and T4 remain normal. Elevated TSH can be another post scarcity effect as the body makes more iodine absorber tissues to absorb the new bounty of iodine supplementation. Your doctor should read Dr. Jorge Flechas' article, *Orthoiodosupplementation in a primary care practice,* especially paragraph five:

www.Optimox.com/pics/Iodine/IOD-10/IOD_10.htm.

The ATP Cofactors have also been used to help TSH return to normal levels.

Iodine cured my painful breasts. But as soon as my family doctor saw my TSH lab tests, he prescribed thyroid hormone and now my painful breasts are back. What happened?

We hear this report occasionally, that prescribing thyroid hormones brings the fibrocystic breast disease back. It appears that prescribing extra thyroid meds speeds up the metabolism of the thyroid, making it need more iodine. So the thyroid, the master regulator, may "steal" the iodine in the bloodstream that had been happily going to the breasts. Dr. Flechas has reported a study of long-term thyroid med takers where they tend to get more breast cancer (Kapdi and Wolfe, 1976). These women were not taking iodine to support the increased metabolism, of course, and one study is not conclusive.

It raises the possibility of the iodine-stealing theory when we see painful breasts return once they're exposed to too much thyroid hormone and not enough iodine. The trick is trying to get a true picture of your thyroid status from an experienced Iodine Literate Practitioner.

More Iodine Stories

Meet Violet, breast cancer survivor:
New breast calcifications (often a precursor to breast cancer) resolve.

On my recent trip to central Australia I took iodine drops with me.

I have been avoiding a mammogram due to the pain factor, around my ex-tumor bed. I was thinking of having an MRI but as I have had dreadful reactions to anesthetic pharmaceuticals in general, and breakout in a rash from something as simple as a bandaid. The thought of being injected with gadolinium scared me off the MRI. My oncologist totally understood.

I haven't had a mammogram since around May 2009. My right breast had quite a few clustered calcifications. Late last year my BS sent me a letter, concerning my mammo appointment that I had been avoiding.

Anyway, I caved in because I understand that clustered calcifications are seen both in benign and malignant disease. So I had my ever sooo painful mammo, which was a tad different to the way I was last examined. The tech actually stayed in the room, and didn't leave. Anyway, we got to chatting and she allowed me to view my breast images on the large computer screen. Cool!

I said, "They look particularly clean, in both breasts; I can't see anything sinister, like calcifications, can you?"

She said, "No, it all looks very clean to me. It appears that the calcifications have all disappeared."

She then said, "Wait here, I'll see what the radiologist thinks." I had my fingers crossed and a huge grin.

They both came back and said. "There's no evidence of calcifications, we'll pass these images on to your oncologist, and I'm sure his conclusion will be the same."

IT WAS!!! He said both breasts were crystal clear ... no problems whatsoever.

My protocol is working for me.

Thank you to *BreastCancerChoices.org* for their wonderful "Iodine resources"... Thank you from the bottom of my heart ... xxxxx.

Meet Ronnie: Varicose veins and broken capillaries healing.

Not only have varicose veins started to go away, I have a tiny patch of broken capillaries on my chin that is now disappearing. I've had them since I was in my twenties due to an injury.

Chapter Eleven

FAQ 7
Iodine Online Discussion Groups

Where can I find online iodine discussion groups?
Each online group pursues iodine information with a different slant, reflecting the varying views of the moderators. Below is a list of the most active groups.

The Iodine Workshop Facebook group focuses on the original protocol which came out of the 2007 Iodine Conferences. Both Dr. David Brownstein's book, *Iodine: Why You Need It*, and this book, *The Iodine Crisis*, are the foundation for the discussion. The group is moderated by iodine pioneer and research editor of *IodineReseach.com*, Lynn Razaitis. Go to: *www.facebook.com/groups/IodineWorkshop*

As of this printing in 2015, over a hundred new cases of life-changing improvements have been reported on the Iodine Workshop. From patients reporting their 20 years of fibromyalgia and brain fog gone, to a cardiac patient now off all drugs with her cardiologist's approval, to a patient with two brain previous brain surgeries from Cushing's disease now in remission—the reports keep coming.

The Curezone Iodine Forum is currently managed by two of its original founders, Laura and Steve. They have had over

10,000,000 hits! The Curezoners offer a deep perspective on how iodine works biochemically and ways it can be used for various ailments. Also, the Curezone Iodine Forum will make a great historical record when someone studies the Grass Roots Iodine Movement. Laura has sleuthed down countless historic documents and photos on iodine found nowhere else in the world. There are many iodine experts on Curezone who have followed iodine supplementation and research for five years or more. The Curezoners have experimented with most every iodine product and reported the results. Several iodine babies have been born— very smart and alert tykes! Go to their website:

http://Curezone.org/forums/f.asp?f=815.

Breast Cancer Think Tank discusses iodine as one aspect of breast healing strategies. The Think Tank is the group I manage. Iodine is discussed as part of a comprehensive breast healing strategy. Link to the group homepage:

http://Health.Groups.yahoo.com/group/breastcancerthinktank.

Other online groups may have good iodine discussions, but the two principal groups are the only two I can personally vouch for as informed and experienced.

More Iodine Stories

Meet Suzanne: Forty years of psoriasis disappears.

When I was diagnosed with breast cancer, my integrative physician put me on Iodoral to prevent recurrence. After a few months, I noticed a case of psoriasis which I've had since puberty disappeared. How did this happen? My mother took me to doctors for years to try and get rid of this disease. Our family spent a fortune on a dozen different treatments. I'm shocked that I had to get breast cancer and discover Iodoral to get rid of the psoriasis.

Meet Wanda, suffering from painful fibrocystic breasts.

A subject I take very seriously. Two years ago, I was well on my way to Breast Cancer. I'd had fibrocystic breast disease (FBD) for a long time; FBD is very much a precursor to breast cancer. By the way, some 90 percent of American women have FBD, NOW. It manifests as lumps and/or breast tenderness, can be cyclical (with the menstrual period), in advanced stages, one can have pain throughout the month.

So, I discovered iodine supplementation. The results have been amazing. I lost a full cup size of painful, swollen tissue. The texture of my breasts completely changed; they have become very soft. I'm 95 percent done; I don't know if the last remaining area is scar tissue, or not. I haven't been diligent about supplementing for a while, now, I've gotten complacent and cocky. So, I need to get back onboard with this.

Chapter Twelve

FAQ 8
Why Is Bromine Dangerous
to Your Health?

*Reminder: since most readers of this book are not chemists,
consider the terms iodine and iodide interchangeable, unless
the difference is relevant to the discussion such as the iodide
in iodized salt.*

*Similarly, the reader should consider the terms bromine and
bromide interchangeable as we discuss the power of any
bromine-related chemical to inhibit iodine.*

What does bromine have to do with iodine deficiency?

Iodine deficiency may be partly a bromide dominance disease,
meaning an underlying cause of iodine deficiency may be that
we are exposed to so much bromine-related chemicals through
baked goods, fire retardants and pesticides, and other hidden
sources. Bromine has bullied what little iodine we have in our
diet off the receptors.

What is bromide dominance?

A bromide dominance condition may develop when bromide,
acquired through environmental, occupational, iatrogenic or

---

dietary exposure, causes bromine levels in the body to rise high enough to inhibit iodine enzyme metabolism.

Iodine supplementation alters the competitive bromine-iodine relationship, causing bromide excretion. Thus, bromide dominance is diminished and proper iodine enzyme metabolism may be restored.

What in my environment contains bromine?

In my opinion, the worst exposure to bromine comes from brominated fire retardant chemicals called BFRs. They are located in rugs, cars, mattresses, upholstery, electronics, children's pajamas, draperies and other items including children's toys. Bromide dust drifts out of the items, is inhaled and gets into our bloodstream.

I read labels. How am I exposed to bromide in foods?

Bromated flour is the norm in baked goods as a dough conditioner. Unless the label specifically reads "unbromated flour," assume the flour is bromated. A local baker told me she was unable to obtain unbromated commercial flour. Look for bromide on labels as "BVO," which stands for brominated vegetable oil. Some sodas and sports drinks contain bromide. Mountain Dew is the best known beverage for containing brominated vegetable oil (BVO).

If you have ordinary toast with breakfast, a sandwich and Mountain Dew for lunch, and then drink a brominated sports drink after your five o'clock jog, you have medicated yourself all day long with bromine and helped purge iodine from your tissues.

See Part 4. *Resources*, for more bromine sources.

If bromine/bromide chemicals are so bad, why aren't they banned by the FDA?

A representative of the FDA told Breast Cancer Choices it doesn't consider bromide a problem.

However, bromide is banned in many countries. The UK banned bromate in bread in 1990. Canada banned bromate in bread in 1994. Sweden is particularly aggressive in banning bromide fire retardants. Since the ban, much less bromide is measured in mothers' milk in Sweden. Some states are trying to ban brominated fire retardants, and the major mattress companies are changing their manufacturing to accommodate demand for less toxic mattresses.

If I just avoid bromide in foods and sodas, do I still need iodine?

Even if you don't consume bromides by mouth or in asthma inhalers, brominated fire retardants from cars, electronics, upholstery, mattresses and carpet are still unavoidable.

Does bromine affect fertility?

Couples with the highest amount of brominated fire retardants in their bloodstream have been reported to have the most infertility problems.

Can bromide affect the sex of my baby?

According to the July 2008 edition of *Environmental Health*, brominated fire retardants (PBDEs) are similar to PCBs which have been demonstrated to cause more female children to be born to women with high levels of the chemical. Brominated fire retardants have been much studied as hormone disruptors in adults as well as animals.

Can Brominated Fire Retardants with PBDEs affect my unborn baby?

According to a 2012 study published in the *Environmental Health Perspectives,* lead author Brenda Eskanazi describes clear neuro-developmental delays. "We measured PBDEs both in the mothers during pregnancy and in the children themselves. It shows that there is a relationship of in utero and childhood levels to decrements in fine motor function, attention and IQ."

What do golf courses have to do with bromide exposure?

The pesticide, methylbromide, may be used on grass. This pesticide is banned in many countries. There is a theory that breast cancer rates in Long Island may be so high because of the number of golf courses contaminated with methylbromide over the years.

More Iodine Stories

Meet Ted: Erections and libido change with direct skin application of Lugol's.

By all means, keep ingesting iodine because the inside-out method is very powerful on so many other levels. But the outside-in painting goes direct to the organs in a profound way.

I have painted 20 drops of 5% elemental iodine (Lugols should work too) on one side of the testes and perineum and then the next night, on the other side, making sure that 48 hours separates the same side painting. That way no sunburn effect happens.

A slight burning occurs momentarily when painting takes place, but is very tolerable.

Incredible results occurred regarding erections. Also, the amount of semen increased.

Erections became even more responsive when I added the oral supplements K2 mk4.

When I added 15 mg, the erections improved in a profound way, several minutes after ingesting the K2. The next morning I awoke with a teenage erection that only a morning pee would relieve. Strangely, I had to reduce the K2 mk4 to just 5 mg a night; but I suspect 3 mg or even 1 mg would work for younger people since I am now 56.

I always do the iodine painting at bed time only ...

I take a dropper and fill it up. Drip about 20 drops back into the bottle and to get an idea where 20 drops are on the dropper glass. That way you don't have to sit there and drip 20 drops each time, give or take a few drops.

I load about 20 drops into the dropper and drag the dropper in the middle of the perineum starting near the backside to the front. I quickly take four fingers and spread the Iodine over the entire area which will include the inside of the leg, the perineum and entire side of the testes.

The next night, I do the other side. After 48 hours pass, you get back to the original side you started with.

Of course, I was still taking large amounts of iodine orally also!

I did it every night for a long time. Now I do it a couple of times a month.

Meet Nancy: Endometriosis resolves. Sex life restored.

I'm 34. After using Iodoral (an iodine supplement) for the past 6 months, I have not had any endometriosis pain and my sex life has been restored, after years of misdiagnosis and indifference by many doctors!

Out of desperation, I sought out a holistic/naturopath doctor for help. He tested my iodine levels right away. It only required a simple saliva and urine test. Turns out my iodine levels were LESS than one part per million. I think regular levels for a woman my age were suppose to be around 10 or 12. He immediately put me on a high dosage of Iodoral supplements.

After retesting my iodine periodically, my iodine level went up, and my pain vanished! I now only take one to two supplements a day to maintain and have been pain-free these past 6 months. (I had the other usual hormone related troubles with endometriosis, and they have subsided as well.) I was skeptical but desperate enough to try this.

I hope someone else can benefit from this information. It's such a simple, non-intrusive thing to try. No side effects. Find a naturopath doctor, make sure they can test your iodine levels via the saliva and urine. If they can't do that, then keep looking. It's important to find someone who knows what they are doing. Research the net about iodine deficiency. It is worth your time! I have needlessly suffered from endometriosis symptoms since my early 20s. I was not diagnosed until two or three years ago. I know how disruptive this can be to your life. You MUST check into iodine supplementation. It has been my miracle!

Part 3

Discovering the World's Oldest Medicine

Chapter Thirteen

Where Does Iodine Come From?

*If we knew what it was we were doing, it would not
be called research, would it?*

—Albert Einstein

D r. David Brownstein calls iodine "the most misunderstood
nutrient."

I'll say! How do you learn about something so misunderstood?
Where do you begin? I'd taught sociology and philosophy for a
living but had zero scientific training. Other than retaining a
solid professional ability to conduct research and split hairs, I
was clueless. But I couldn't let being clueless stop me. There
were no textbooks on how to learn about iodine, so I was on my
own whether I liked it or not.

Iodine had become so important to my own health that I
needed to create an expedition to learn about this transforming
element. Where could I start? How much was there to learn, anyway? I tried to remember how I had learned before when I was
out of my depth.

Field Guide? What is a field guide? The answer to this question
came on my eighth summer when my father squeezed us kids
into the car with two weeks' worth of beach gear and handed
me a book called a *Field Guide for Seashore Life*. He knew how to

keep me quiet during the long drive down the Garden State Parkway. Included were terrific pictures and diagrams of how marine life at the shore was set up.

How to observe. How to question. The book gave me a structure for my curiosity. It gave me confidence.

I had never thought of nature as so organized that someone could draw a blueprint of the places where the natural things lived. So, natural things had a home just like people. The best part of the guide was it laid out an actual how-to for collecting and preserving what they called "specimens."—that was the word for the bounty surrounding my bare feet on the sand.

According to the book, conducting a research expedition into the field and finding specimens was the official way of learning. Back then, I didn't know there were actual ways of learning. I thought teachers taught the three Rs. Period. I thought they inserted information into your brain. The authors called it a *field guide* because the emphasis was on throwing the student in the deep end so she could figure out how to learn.

How to observe. How to question. The book gave me a structure for my curiosity. It gave me confidence. You identify your mission and jump into the field. Use binoculars, use a shovel, use a magnifying glass but learn to pry, learn to observe. You can watch others observe but you have to grow your own observation "chops." Otherwise, people will tell you what you see and you'll always see through a second-hand filter.

According to *The Field Guide*, the object was to hunt specimens down, identify them and figure out the story behind them. Wow, that was for me. I wanted to discover how all this ocean stuff fit together. How hard could that be? *The Field Guide* was only about 200 pages.

In retrospect, I had two things going for me that would seed who I am and what I do:

> First, I was young enough to be curious. Learning hadn't been used against me yet in school. I liked being a beginner. Learning was still my fun friend. No one had told me I wasn't qualified to learn by myself.
>
> Second, I owe my parents a debt of gratitude because they just left us kids to learn by ourselves. They got out of our way.

First thing the next morning, I grabbed my yellow pail and shovel and headed off the back porch of our seashore bungalow and headed to the bay in my bathing suit. My mother yelled after me what she and the other moms always yelled when they didn't go with us, "Don't go in the water past your knees."

The Expedition Begins

I walked along the sand in my flip flops, determined to search for these seashore specimen things in the field guide.

I scooped up some shells that looked like slippers and some tiny iridescent disks the size of quarters. I wasn't sure how these things had ever been alive or if they were still alive. The book said to put the specimens in the yellow pail with seawater just in case. But by the time I reached the jetty rocks, I realized my flip flops wouldn't let me climb over the rocks without slipping. I tried anyway but just scuffed my feet.

I ran back home and got my sneakers. I had noticed seaweeds and shells growing on the rocks so I asked for my father's putty knife to pry away specimens. I set out once again to the bay and climbed the rocks with ease, prying off limpets, seaweeds and mussels from the rocks and putting them into my plastic pail. At the cove in the rocks, I discovered a little tide pool with a whole different set of sea life living there. The life under the water looked clean and magnified, larger than life. I jumped in with my sneakers and began picking up specimens and covering them with water just as the book instructed. But my sneakers sloshed and slipped in the calf-high water. Sand got through the canvas and scraped my feet. I couldn't reach the tide pool sea-life with sneakers. I needed boots.

Back to the bungalow I ran, sneakers sloshing, my yellow pail full. "Mom, the sneakers don't work in the water. I'm gonna need boots." My mother laid my sneakers on the porch to dry in the sun and got out my green, frog-eye rain boots. I emptied my pail of slimy specimens into an enamel basin and set it down in the shade under the porch so the specimens wouldn't die.

Down to the bayside I headed again, this time in my bathing suit and rain boots outfit. The tide was going out. I ignored the glances of the other kids and made my way back over the now slimy, low-tide rocks to the tide pool. I jumped into the water with my boots and began scooping as many specimens as I could. But the tide pool was full of so many creatures that I couldn't fit them into the toy pail.

Back to the house I went, sunburn starting on my shoulders. "Lynne, you're getting red. You need Noxema," my mother said, going into the house and returning with a blue jar. She spread the methol cream on my shoulders and face. "That should do it. Are you finished for today?"

"No, Mom, this time I'm gonna need a bigger pail."

She looked concerned. "Bigger pail?" What was I getting into if I needed a bigger pail? She was thinking about the ship captain in *Jaws*. After his first encounter with the Great White shark, he says, "We're gonna need a bigger boat."

Still, she saw my passion. She found an aluminum kitchen pail under the sink and watched me adventure out one more time. By then, the sun had risen high and its light bounced off the water, making it harder to see, so I kept my head down. I didn't want to go back for sunglasses.

Along the bay I walked again, this time smeared with Noxema, boots clopping and grown-up pail swinging. Now I was prepared. Over the rocks I climbed and jumped into the tide pool. Sea gulls screamed overhead, knowing I was competition for their lunch. A scary-looking horseshoe crab scooted away in the water, but I was able to scoop up some fuzzy sea crabs and at least ten different seaweeds, a measled cowrie, Atlantic slipper shells and a whelk egg case. I piled each into my pail and covered them with water so they wouldn't die. They needed to be alive so I could identify them. By the time the aluminum pail was half full, I realized I could barely lift it. I threw some stuff back to lighten the load. But the pail remained heavy.

Crap! Why didn't anyone tell me a full three gallon pail weighs more than an eight year-old can carry? I trod home with my pail only half-full of specimens and a funny green seaweed called Bladderwrack. By the time I reached the porch my arms ached, but frustration had turned to pride. I wasn't about to wait for someone to teach me how to collect specimens or have them carry them home for me. I wasn't going to wait until I knew exactly what I was doing. If I had waited for either skill or strength, I would never have begun or known what I was capable of. The next day I returned from the bay with another half bucket of specimens. And then another. I was in my element.

Every night at the shore, I showed my parents the specimens and repeated the names of each shell or organism. "How do you memorize all the names?" my father asked.

"But I didn't memorize them," I answered. "I just looked them up. All the pictures are right there in the *Field Guide*.

"Good work, Sweetie," he said. "You never know what will come in handy some day."

Another Field Trip, Another Expedition

When Iodine transformed my life decades later, there was no *Field Guide* for researching iodine history. I set out on an expedition with clues but no map, with a few books but no artifacts, with a handful of theories but no case studies. I learned from the old *Merck Manual* that iodine was the most used tumor remedy in the 1800s and a treatment for lung diseases, goiter and even for syphilis. But what about before that?

- Where did iodine come from? Iodine must have left a trail of artifacts and information behind.
- Where did the trail begin?
- When did people first start using iodine products?
- Could I find some of these iodine products the way I had collected specimens from the sea?
- When were seaweeds first recorded?
- If iodine was so important, why was it invisible in my life?
- Iodine wasn't used much as an antiseptic in my generation but I remembered seeing it. Where?

I wracked my brain. My only personal exposure to iodine had been the radioactive dye from the CT scan years ago when I had all those headaches. Then there was some vinyl iodine formulation called Povidone, swabbed on my mother's skin as an antiseptic before a surgery. Where could I look first?

I began the field trip in my own home starting with a dusty bottle of *Tincture of Iodine,* marked with a skull and cross bones, in the back of our family's overflowing, remedy-for-anything medicine cabinet. Nobody knew where it came from. I also found a milk-glass jar of something called Iodex ointment with a label looking like it had been designed in the 1950s. My Swedish mother-in-law, Alfhild, swore by Iodex, rubbing it into bruises and sprains. I only kept it in the cabinet as a keepsake because she was so passionate about her Iodex. Our family medicine chest was all I needed for my first specimens ... Two specimens. Not much. Not even enough to fill a small pail, but it was the first step.

Since I didn't know anything about iodine's beginnings, I could only start at the present and work backward. Was I qualified to do this research? I'd read a book titled *The Historian as Detective* in graduate school. It encouraged students to do history by collecting "primary sources" and not to accept any common hearsay history because it was riddled by bias and the current groupthink. "History," Mr. Sawyer, my high school history teacher told us, "often records only a few events in the lives of great men, not the events around them."

By great, he meant heads of state, generals, officials in charge. By men he meant, well, *males*. The rest of the culture was relegated to the margins. Paradoxically, how the majority of the people lived was considered such insignificant historical information that it was pushed off into sociology and anthropology, the so-called sideline, "squint" disciplines.

The Plan

Howard Zinn's *A Peoples' History of the United States* also encourages readers to excavate and sieve through what they find, to tell an original story. Independent scholars often access information that the rank and file historians miss because they are unshackled by the premises of the status quo. Was I qualified to pursue the history of iodine? There was no way of knowing what the qualifications were since nobody else had done it. No one knew where the beginning began.

Since there was no known history of iodine, I decided to work my way backwards from my own medicine cabinet to the healers of centuries past. I would need to reverse-engineer the journey from the present, backwards in time, to discover eras when iodine was used abundantly. Maybe then I could explore the mystery of why iodine had gone missing during my lifetime.

In 2005, I prepared to be a student again. I prepared for an expedition into iodine's history. I used the tools that I had learned as a kid: Read what you can find in the conventional literature. Then, open your eyes and look outside the box. Get away from groupthink. Find actual evidence the way the *Field Guide* instructed me to learn by digging up specimens and examining them. Get your feet wet and hands dirty, just like those days long ago at the shore:

- Prehistoric finds
- Ancient Chinese cure books
- Egyptian Papyrus
- Pharmacy records
- Antique medical preparations
- Advertising flyers
- Personal letters
- Iodine lockets
- Iodine prostate suppositories
- Inhalers
- Breast ointments from 1900

All these helped me construct a history of how iodine was used, first as a seaweed medicine, then a pharmaceutical.

I begin at the current known beginning, 15,000 years ago, but future anthropologists will no doubt excavate even older evidence of the world's oldest medicine.

More Iodine Stories

Meet John: Increased energy, no migraines since starting Iodoral.

Here's what I can report:

1) Increased mental and physical energy. I had more energy within hours after the first dose.
2) Greatly reduced migraine headaches. I had been bothered with migraines since my early teens but they had reduced in intensity sharply in my late 50s to a mere inconvenience. I haven't really had a headache (that I could identify as a headache) since I started Iodoral just over a year ago.
3) I have tried to get others to try a little IODINE supplementation. None have. I imagine they figure I'm just another "vitamin nut."

Meet Candace: Depression, lethargy, puffy face resolve.

I work as a nurse in an osteopathic physician's office. I'm 24 and was very depressed and lethargic. I watched TV in my apartment every night. I kept going by drinking coffee. Then I saw the doctor was prescribing a lot of iodine in his practice and the patients were improving. So I tried it on my own. It changed my life. I've lost 30 pounds and a lot of puffiness has left my face. I'm now dating and don't understand what was wrong with me that iodine fixed. The doctor thinks it may have been my thyroid or adrenals. I don't really care. I always panic if I think I may run out of iodine. I don't want that person I used to be.

Meet Samantha: Uterine fibroids, fibrocystic breast disease, not detectible after nine months.

I am one of those people who have had great success with iodine supplementation to cure uterine fibroids. I use Lugol's solution, as it has more elemental iodine than plain SSKI which is just potassium iodide. Elemental iodine is really important for women with uterine fibroids or fibrocystic breast disease (which I also had).

I started with 50 mg Lugols per day (6-8 drops) in a glass of water, first thing in the morning. I did have a week or so of detox reaction, but upped the dose to 100mg per day, and these detox symptoms passed quickly. In a few weeks I saw dramatic reduction in my FBD, and the uterine fibroids started shrinking.

After six months of iodine supplementation most of the FBD was gone, and the uterine fibroids were almost gone.

After nine months, I had a breast examination and no FBD could be detected at all, I also had an ultrasound and no uterine fibroids could be detected either. My cycle is now normal, with no pain, and regular as clockwork.

Meet Deiter: Atrial fibrillation improvement. No more herpes lip flare-ups.

I have been gradually but cautiously increasing number of drops of 5% Lugols, now on four drops per day. I've gained over ten pounds, I try liver detox and use the Magnesium/Salt/Vita C/water/protocol. Only thing I have noticed is a smoother heartbeat, less A-fib episodes and no herpes lip flare-ups. My beard seems fuller.

Meet Donna: Energy returns. PMS fatigue gone.

I decided to up my Iodoral intake to the full pill from half, for the long weekend off from work. Well, the difference in my energy is astounding. I have accomplished a huge amount in my home in the last two days plus got the shopping done and am taking care of a very sick husband.

I am also in the middle of PMS week, which normally means I would lay around and get nothing done.

I am going to stay at this level for at least a week and then go up another half a pill. I'm not sure I'll ever go as high as 50 mg, but you never know.

Meet Holly: Dry eyes and vaginal dryness helped by iodine.

I recently had a two week break from iodine for various (life craziness) reasons ... and while I never noticed dry eyes before I started the iodine, I could REALLY notice the difference during the time I was off iodine.

My eyes were dry and somewhat itchy. I started up the iodine again and after a couple of days my eyes returned to normal. I meant to post about it here and totally forgot (see, I really should be better at taking my iodine! As soon as I stop, my mind and body fall apart)

I also notice vaginal dryness when not taking iodine.

I recall watching a video link a while back about how iodine affects the body, and it is important for any organ/gland that secretes ... so that actually fits, if you think about it. Our eyes constantly need to secrete tiny amounts of fluid to stay lubricated. I don't know how or why, but somehow iodine helps with maintaining secretion throughout the body.

Chapter Fourteen

The Buried History of Iodine

In solving a problem of this sort, the grand thing is to be able to reason backwards. That's a very useful accomplishment, and a very easy one, but people do not practice it much.

—Sherlock Holmes
in Sir Arthur Conan Doyle's A Study in Scarlet

The history of iodine is too colorful and complex to lay out in a linear, this-came-first, this-came-next, fashion. There are too many intersecting stories that encompass wars, from the Napoleonic to the Vietnam, too many stories that encompass medical rivalries, wild bootlegging and heartbreaking cases of mental retardation. Iodine has been used on Civil War battle-fields and painted onto swollen breasts. Nobody understands exactly how iodine works but its historical record is "writ" large. Readers will judge how iodine's long history validates our respect for the violet colored element. I'll hit on the history parts that moved me. Take what you want and leave the rest. I've put a timeline at the end for those not keen on stories.

Before iodine was identified as an element in 1811, the world's oldest nutrient was found in its most concentrated form in seaweeds. Algae, another term for seaweed, is believed to be the first anti-oxidant from an evolutionary perspective.

If we go back to prehistoric times, archaeological excavation tells the story of how iodine-rich seaweeds were used as both food and medicines. Archaeological sites reveal exactly how healers practiced seaweed medicine. Its use stretches into the far distant past:

- Long before iodine was isolated and discovered as an element in 1811;
- Before the 1811 French records showing iodine was extracted from seaweed;
- Before the 3000 year-old Chinese Herbal manual, *Pen Tsao*;
- Before the Egyptian *Ebers' Medical Papyrus*; and
- Before the recorded Auyurvedic Medicine of India.

Digging up a 15,000 Year-Old Seaweed Medicine Hut

In 1975, a veterinary student from the Southern University of Chile stumbled on what he thought was a cow bone while out for a walk. His discovery turned out to be a mastodon tusk and contained scrape marks where humans had cut away the meat. This finding launched a 10 year excavation project by archaeologist Tom Dillehay and his colleagues. They dug and they dug. They picked at the fibers in the soil with dental picks. They sifted, they radiocarbon dated and then dug some more. What they discovered was a roughly 15,000 year-old site containing a small village of huts.

Nine seaweed species were found among the plant and animal remains. When the scientists examined the material microscopically, they found all nine species were excellent sources of iodine, zinc, hormones and trace elements, as well as protein. Archaeologists who specialize in the analysis of plants to discover how ancient societies organized themselves, participate in the specialized field of *archeobotany*. They discovered that those prehistoric people consumed seaweeds which regulated cholesterol metabolism, strengthened bones and strengthened immune response. The findings show how sophisticated the prehistoric people were with respect to plant medicine.

One of the Monte Verde, Chile village structures was set apart as a "medicine hut" where the seaweeds were prepared. Some specimens were found dried, showing they had been preserved, and some specimens were burnt in the way later healers used to use seaweed ashes to treat goiter. Eventually the iodine component of seaweed was identified by the researchers as the most active ingredient. What archaeologists called a "masticated cud" with antibiotic properties was found with teeth marks, suggesting one of the ways seaweed was consumed was in the form of a large lozenge that would get the medicine directly into the bloodstream via the blood vessels in the mouth, bypassing digestion.

It is known that iodine in its isolated form can irritate the stomach. One might speculate this lozenge may have been designed to eliminate the problem; the same problem Dr. Guy Abraham solved 15,000 years later by coating his iodine tablets with a pharmaceutical glaze so they wouldn't irritate the stomach . . . Caveman, meet Dr. A.

Another striking discovery about the prehistoric Monte Verde inhabitants is that they lived in a region rich with plants and animals, but seaweeds were not available locally. The nearest seaweeds came from the far distant coast. Natives would have needed to walk 90 kilometers west to acquire it from the seacoast or else find prehistoric trading partners. This information shows how prized seaweeds were to their culture.

From Prehistoric Chile to Vitamin Shoppe

According to Dillehay's supporting materials for *Monte Verde: Seaweed, Food, Medicine, and the Peopling of South America*, some of the excavated seaweeds are still used today by the indigenous

Huilliche people to treat rashes, inflammations, abscesses, tumors, ulcers, eye infections, gout and other conditions. I found Gigartina, one of the seaweeds found at the Monte Verde site, in capsules in the Vitamin Shoppe chain store. Research shows this red seaweed has been used for millennia as an immune stimulant and antiviral in traditional Chinese medicine as well as other cultures. Many contemporary naturopaths and herbalists recommend Gigartina, unaware that 15,000 years ago prehistoric peoples used the exact same botanical.

Fast forward ten centuries. Written history actually documents seaweeds as medicine. Herbal medicine books were among the first books produced, written by hand, in ancient China, Egypt, India and Europe. Most often such writings were created on manuscript "paper" or scrolls and recorded the traditional medical practices. They were often accompanied by drawings so the reader could identify the right plant.

The Emperor Shennong is credited with the founding of Chinese herbal medicine, but most likely he only possessed the foresight to record traditional remedies which had been passed along by word of mouth through the generations. They were recorded in the *Pen Ts'ao ching* or *Great Herbal* pharmacopoeia in about 2700 BCE. Hai Tsao, one of the seaweeds found at the Monte Verde site, also is listed in the ancient Chinese herbal as a treatment for tumors, goiter and tuberculosis. Laminaria, a brown seaweed, was recommended for tumors then and is still studied by scientists 3,000 years later.

The famous Ebers Medical Papyrus was reportedly found between the legs of a mummy in an Egyptian burial ground. When the 110 page scroll was finally translated into English by an Egyptian endocrinologist in 1987, the manuscript revealed that the Egyptians used seaweeds for breast tumors. The ancient Indian Ayurvedic medicine employed seaweed as well. The

Materia Medica, a compilation of medical remedies, reports the same information, showing seaweed was a universally known remedy for everything from tumors to parasites for millennia.

Goiter was sometimes referred to as "fat neck." Hippocrates, the ancient Greek philosopher known as the father of Western medicine, widely known for authoring the oath, "First do no harm," also prescribed seaweed. Hippocrates made medicine a discipline distinct from philosophy but maintained philosophy's imperative to look for errors in reasoning within medicine. He urged meticulous documenting of all clinical observations as well as taking elaborate case histories of the whole person. These holistic practices, which were the standard of care in Ancient Greece, mostly died out after his death. But at least he passed on the tradition of treating the thyroid with seaweed to his many followers.

Later, in the 1st century AD, naturalist Pliny the Elder recommended copious burnt seaweed as a sure remedy for "neck swelling." In the Middle Ages there is some reference to the healers Galen and Avicenna, recommending the same remedy. So it's hard to know if the remedy was discovered in one place and spread, or if it was independently discovered in so many places, seaweeds as medicine were common knowledge in different pockets around the globe.

The Native Healer Known as *Seaweed Man*

Sometimes, western explorers or missionaries stumbled onto seaweed medicine. When the Lutheran missionaries attempted to convert the aboriginal people of Australia in the 1800s, they built a village and tried to "civilize" the natives. But the locals still retained faith in their medicine man—called *"parraitye-orn"*—which translated into "seaweed man."

But seaweed knowledge eluded some. When British whaling ships went out on expeditions lasting as long as three years, they would often report with disgust that some primitive peoples ate seaweed. As many as a third of the whalers died of scurvy, unaware that vitamin C was there for the taking in the seaweed floating around their ship.

More Iodine Stories

Meet Brittany: Severe fibromyalgia pain and fatigue resolve.

I'm a 28 year–old woman with three active kids. I developed fibromyalgia in my upper back after the birth of my first child in 2003. The pain and spasms progressed into deep throbbing pain within three years and after my second child. Spasms have gotten so bad and so frequent that I fear them. The longest one lasted 14 hours and put me in the ER. When it was over, I threw up everywhere, slept for a week and lost 10 pounds. My most recent spasm was about 6 months ago. They tend to last about two to three hours but can last longer. Sometimes I went months without them and then there are months I have them every week. When I say spasms, think of having the wind knocked out of you while being crushed by a truck and someone twisting a knife in and out of your shoulder blade. It was that bad. I felt like a 70 year-old trapped in a thirty-year old body.

My fatigue was so severe, I fell asleep while driving. As soon as I got up in the morning, putting on clothes was a chore. Even though I had love in my life, and children and a wonderful husband, I don't understand how I lived so many years feeling so miserable and NO ONE HELPED ME! Doctors are so careless! I gained 20 pounds in six months doing nothing different. My skin was getting bad. Dry but breaking out.

I had to take Tramodol prescription pain killer. Then, in looking up fibromyalgia on the web, I came across iodine as a therapy.

It seemed cheap enough, so the first thing I did was apply some Lugol's Iodine to my foot. Then I started taking it orally. Everything changed. One day I realized I forgot to take my pain meds.

Within two weeks of starting iodine, I feel like I have gotten my life back. I feel ashamed to have lived in a stupor like a zombie for so long, just trying to get by each day. Even in the midst of detox symptoms, I have done more in two weeks than I have in the last year! I feel awesome! I LOVE life! I am losing inches, not weight yet, but who cares!? I have apologized profusely to my husband for being so sick and lazy and thanked him for loving me so much. He basically took care of me and three kids for the last three years as I had been progressively getting worse.

Even though I am so happy now, I want to cry for my old self and the years wasted. I want to help those around me. I see obese women and tired men and feel so bad for them. I want to help! I'm awake and alive! I'm even smarter. Now I realize that it is not healthy to accept life-deteriorating health just due to aging. A 60-year-old shouldn't have ever felt the way I did.

Are there any other young moms out there who can relate to my story? My doctor also gave me anti-anxiety meds and wanted to put me on antidepressants.

Now I come home from work and get right down to making dinner for the family. I now have so much energy I could make two dinners every night!

Meet Sonja: Bleeding gums resolve.

My greatest iodine success is curing long-time bleeding gums. I had irritated gums between two teeth for over a year, even with the gentlest flossing. My dentist did what she could, but my gums didn't heal. I got a prescription mouthwash—which I used for two months without it helping at all. I even thought at some time that my tooth may have a hidden crack because of the pain.

After a while, I thought about trying Lugol's 5% on the problem area. Just one drop mornings and evenings after flossing. After one week, I was significantly better. I found expanding floss which, after a little use, lost the original waxing of the thread. I then soaked part of the floss and used it once more between in the problem areas. After just one more week, the gums had healed and were healthy once more—after well over a year of suffering. I've stopped the iodine treatment (the iodine flossing) and now just take my iodine the regular way—2 drops in water in the morning and one drop in the evening. I sometimes swish the solution, but I don't do any topical treatment any more. And my gums are still healthy.

I still keep up the iodine (+ selenium). I have Hashimoto's and have not registered any adverse effect of iodine. My TSH may have increased a little, but so have fT4 and fT3 (so much for the "reliable TSH"!) and my energy levels.

Chapter Fifteen

A Magic Purple Haze—
Iodine Emerges from the Ashes—
Its Discovery as an Element

We shall not cease from exploration
And the end of all our exploring
Will be to arrive where we started
And know the place for the first time.

—T.S. Eliot, Four Quartets

No one could invent a story as magical as the true story. The discovery of iodine as a life-changing chemical element happened the way a magician pours a mysterious liquid into a top hat and then, in a cloud of sparkles, poof, pulls out a white rabbit. For years, medicine had known seaweed had healing powers but nobody knew why. Then in 1811, a chemical accident transformed Western medicine.

French chemist Bernard Courtois had worked in the family manufacturing business in Dijon making saltpeter, an ingredient used to make gunpowder for Napolean's wars. One day Courtois ran out of the customary wood ash, so he acquired seaweed which was abundant on the shores of Normandy and Brittany.

He burned seaweed in a copper vessel, and then accidentally poured too much sulfuric acid onto the ashes. Whoosh, a beautiful violet vapor emerged. The vapor crystallized into a luminous powder the color of graphite.

Then and there, Courtois suspected he had discovered a new element but was too poor to experiment, so he gave his wealthier chemist friends samples of the crystals for experimentation. He didn't realize that extra sulfuric acid created one of the most fortuitous accidents in medical history.

Two years later, Humphrey Davy sent a letter to the Royal Society of London naming the new element *Iodes*, the Greek word for violet. Later in the 1800s, many scientific "fathers" claimed a role in iodine's conception. Courtois, who launched the revolution of scientific discovery died penniless because he didn't register his discovery.

In the next few years, iodine was picked up by physicians for the treatment of many diseases. Since burnt seaweed and sea sponges had often been used to treat goiter for thousands of years, doctors in England and Europe began to make the connection that it was actually the iodine in these sea plants that shrunk the sick, swollen thyroids of goiter. Word spread fast. Thousands of articles were published. Reports documented too many diseases to count with accuracy in the following years.

1820 to 1900—Iodine Goes Viral

Lung diseases were the scourge of Europe in the 1900s. Patients who had often recovered by surrounding their hospital beds with seaweed, now took iodine.

In 1829, Jean Lugol, a Paris doctor, first invented a popular iodine formulation known as Lugol's Solution which contained 5% iodine and 10% potassium iodide mixed with distilled water. It was first created for the lungs, but over the years, it has been used for everything from purifying water to treating thyroid conditions. As the 1800s passed, iodine became what has been called "the Swiss Army Knife of Medicine."

According to Francis C. Kelly, writing in the Proceedings of the Royal Society of Medicine, 1961, "The variety of diseases for which iodine was prescribed in the early years is astonishing—paralysis, chorea, scrofula, lacrimal fistula, deafness, distortions of the spine, hip joint disease, syphilis, acute inflammation, gout, gangrene, dropsy, carbuncles, whitlow, chilblains, burns, scalds, croup, catarrh, asthma, ulcers and bronchitis—to mention only a few." He reports there that between 1820 and 1840, many publications appeared documenting the various applications.

Albert Szentgorgi, the 1937 Nobel Prize winner credited with the discovery of Vitamin C, claimed doctors in his era had a saying about potassium iodide (KI):

If you know not where or why, use you then K and I.

We often forget that syphilis infected 50 percent of Europe in the late 1800s. When Van Gogh contracted syphilis, he wrote a letter to his brother, Theo, on how iodine helped the brain and the spine. We don't know what form he used in turn-of-the-century France, but we do know Bismuth Formic Iodide Compound was available at American pharmacies to combat syphilitic lesions. Toxic mercury was used until it was replaced by potassium iodide in 1840 for the later stages of syphilis and was used until 1929 when Penicillin was invented. In reviewing pharmacy ledgers from that era, I found thousands of iodine-based compounds prescribed by doctors for lesions.

1800s The Breasts Love Iodine

Doctors advised women to paint their painful and cystic breasts with iodine. Some breast cancer doctors injected iodine directly into the breasts or ovaries for swelling and cysts. Iodine was used in hundreds of breast cancer case studies reported by famed surgeon Dr. Alfred Valpeau in his *A Treatise on Cancer of the Breast and of the Mammary Region (1856)*.

You would think the records of disease and treatments would be presented in a dry or academic fashion. But 150 years ago, case studies were written up with meticulous and compassionate care. Doctors reflected on their options and shared both their optimism and restraint, their enthusiasm and disappointment. An iodine medical industry grew, developing new ways to administer iodine. Many drug companies developed their own formulations combining iodine with other elements.

Patients caught on and reported their successes. In collecting artifacts and iodine memorabilia for the Breast Cancer Choices research project, I purchased an antique letter for sale, dated May 31, 1886. Addressed to "Mrs. Dr. R. A. Johnston" in Wellsville, Ohio, it came from her sister. The letter writer described how she had successfully relieved pain by painting iodine on her breast the way the doctor's wife had recommended. What is significant is that this letter provided insight into successful patient-to-patient medicine in the late 1800s, and that the many monographs and books published by medical doctors on iodine and the breast did not constitute fad, hype or hyperbole. The patients reported success to each other.

The American Civil War—The Iodine Cure for Cannonballs

In 2006, while cruising eBay for iodine artifacts, I stumbled on a brass iodine canteen with markings indicating it was used by the Confederate soldiers during the Civil War. I later discovered soldiers carried iodine canteens along with water canteens as an essential part of their pack. Iodine was used to purify water and to treat infections from unsanitary conditions or even the complications of battlefield surgeries and gunshot wounds. Long after I had snared the canteen for Breast Cancer Choices' iodine artifact collection, I read the report by Francis Kelly of a Confederate soldier who might have used such a canteen.

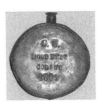

**Figure 4
Confederate States Civil
War Iodine Canteen,
1861.** (Collection of Breast
Cancer Choices.)

Kelly recalls the story of a Confederate Colonel, John B. Gordon, who sustained several cannonball injuries to his leg, arm, shoulder and face. Infection set in. When he was removed to a hospital, Dr. Weatherly of the 6th Alabama Regiment prescribed Tincture of Iodine applied to the wounds three or four times a day. Gordon claims his wife may have misunderstood the instructions and applied the iodine three or four hundred times a day. The Colonel not only recovered, be went on to become Governor of Georgia and lived a long life. He died in 1904, forty years after his Civil War experience.

Soldiers carried iodine canteens along with water canteens as an essential part of their pack.

129

Iodine: The Infection Connection

Today we know that iodine's effects are broader than its antiseptic properties. We have learned that it detoxifies metals, strengthens the endocrine system and has unexplained mechanisms of action in the brain and other body systems.

At the turn of the 20th century, iodine was so popular for lung diseases, that medical catalogs featured elaborate devices called nebulizers; they were intended to promote inhalation according to certain documented protocols. Iodine sometimes drove toxins from the lungs so powerfully that care was needed to slow down the detoxification process. Dr. Abraham uses the word, "deobstruent," to describe the process of driving toxins and impurities from the blood and tissues. Iodine was widely believed to prevent viral infection. The British Red Cross even manufactured lockets embedded with iodine-soaked cotton.

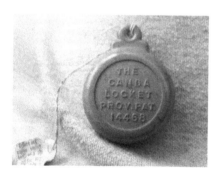

Figure 5
Red Cross Iodine Locket embedded with iodine-soaked cotton.
(Collection of Breast Cancer Choices.)

Iodizing Salt Takes 100 Years (no, that's not a typo)

Even though French nutritional chemist Jean-Baptiste Bousingalt had recommended adding **iodine to salt** in 1830s, it took Dr. David Marine until 1924 to get salt iodized in the United States. He achieved this feat by creating an experiment on adolescents from Akron, Ohio, where the soil was notoriously iodine deficient. Goiter affected 56 percent of the population and girls were six times more likely to develop goiter than boys. Researchers took approximately 2,000 pupils and gave them iodide. The control group of approximately the same number of pupils received no iodide. After 30 months, 22 percent of the students not given iodide developed goiter. Only two percent of the students receiving iodide developed goiter.

In less than ten years after salt was iodized, goiter incidence plummeted. In Detroit, goiter rates dropped from 9.7 percent to 1.4 percent in the first six years of using iodized salt.

Soldier, Your Neck Is Too Fat

Scholars such as Quynh Nguyen observed, in *Iodized Salt and US Development*, that before the iodization of salt, the US Army rejected many "Goiter Belt" recruits for significant goiter. During the First World War nearly 12,000 men had simple goiter and one third of those were rejected because their necks were so large the military shirts' collars could not be fastened. Even soldiers accepted into the army tended to have larger necks than soldiers elsewhere and needed larger shirts. After salt iodization, fewer Goiter Belt recruits were rejected and the Army began making shirts with smaller collars.

By the 1900s the benefits of iodine as an important nutrient even penetrated rural communities of South Carolina. There they were so proud of their iodine-rich soil they marketed bootleg liquor with the slogan, "Not a goiter in a gallon." In order to further advertise their healthy produce, SOUTH CAROLINA, THE IODINE STATE, was stamped on license plates.

But not every place in the world is lucky enough to have a Seaweed Man as the local healer or a state as rich in iodine soil as South Carolina. Many countries and areas are devastated by iodine deficiency. In 1996, China was estimated to have ten million people suffering from mental retardation because of iodine deficiency in the soil.

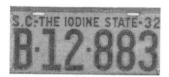

Figure 6
1932 South Carolina
License Plate, *The*
Iodine State.
(Collection of Breast
Cancer Choices.)

In 1989, when pediatric neurologist Dr. G. Robert DeLong of Duke University Medical School first visited the rural Chinese province Xinjiang , mental retardation was severe. Other disabilities also prevailed: miscarriages, high infant mortality, stunted growth, deafness and stillbirths affected much of the population.

Some of the fully developed adults appeared as small as children. Some of the five year-olds looked like toddlers. According to DeLong, the children were truly in sad shape. "Some showed extreme mental retardation and could not walk, stand or even sit. Even the ones without severe signs of physical debilitation were slack and dull-eyed."

Their livestock were similarly feeble and produced stillborn offspring, leaving the province desperately poor. Since this area of China had been regarded as inhabited by "village idiots" since Marco Polo's time in the 1200s, the people had been "written off." Iodized salt was not an option because of many cultural and political factors including fear of the salt.

Dr. DeLong and his colleagues in China explored and rejected many solutions for getting iodine into the people. Finally, DeLong looked at the irrigation ditches and wondered if iodine could be dripped into the water. That way the plants would absorb the iodine, the animals would eat the plants and the people on top of the food chain would get enough iodine.

How did they do this? They had to be practical. Think low tech. DeLong and his Chinese colleagues rigged a common 55 gallon oil drum on top of a rickety bridge that crossed the irrigation canal. They attached some intravenous tubing and clamps to provide a steady drip into the water. Next, they filled the drum with potassium iodate and measured how much iodine turned up in the downstream villages. When they were ready, they hired a local villager to guard the barrel from theft. At night he slept on the bridge, rolled up in a blanket. As the iodine ran out, the villagers continued to refill the barrels.

Figure 7
Xinjiang Provence villager guards barrel used to drip iodine into the irrigation ditch.
(Photo courtesy of Shannon Hader.)

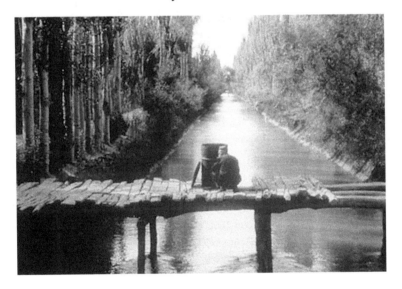

How to Drop Infant Mortality by Half

A year later,

- Infant mortality dropped by half.
- Sheep production increased 40 percent.

- Later measurements showed the average five-year-old's height increased by four inches.
- The average intelligence of children born after the irrigation project increased 16 IQ points.
- Stillborn animals and miscarriage were reduced by 50 percent.

By 1997, The Thrasher Foundation, The Joseph P. Kennedy Foundation and Kiwanis International jumped in to underwrite the irrigation project. Iodine dripping is now implemented for 2.6 million Chinese. Thirteen and one-half tons of iodine have been dripped into the villagers' water. The cost for such a life saving, life altering project? Less than six cents per person. That's all it cost to rewrite the lives of people who had been written off for five centuries.

In Kazakhstan, a country located in Central Asia, public health officials try hard to raise awareness about the importance of iodine to intelligence. Billboards shout out the iodine message. Pamphlets are distributed and studied by seventh graders. Even the *Iodine Man* super hero cartoon character urges children not to be stupid; "eat iodized salt." Even with all these educational tools, Valentina Sivryukova, president of the national confederation of Kazakh charities, was never sure the message got through until, while walking through the market one day, she heard one young Kazakh boy tease another, calling out, "What are you, iodine-deficient or something?"

What Difference Does 15 IQ Points Make?

In Zaire, public health workers travelled to remote areas where mental retardation was so devastating that they felt the best way to get iodine into the population was to inject them with iodine in a base of poppy seed oil. In one case, an adult man whose IQ was estimated to be in the 50s, was so mentally impaired from iodine deficiency, that he didn't understand he needed to wear clothes. His aging parents were so ashamed that they had to keep him locked in the house so as not to upset the villagers. After the public health workers gave him an injection of iodine mixed with poppy seed oil, he learned to keep his clothes on and was able to get a job loading bricks onto a truck. This not only helped the family finances but their status in their village. The parents were among many who walked many miles to thank the public health workers for changing their lives.

Unfortunately, it has been hard to create awareness that iodine is not just a concern for poor countries where mass mental retardation or Cretinism presents a huge health problem. Countries such as India are so serious about the importance of iodized salt that you can go to jail if you're caught transporting or selling contraband uniodized salt.

So here we are at the beginning of the 21st century. If iodine deficiency is the leading cause of mental retardation and if iodine can reverse breast disease and many other medical conditions, why don't we know more about it? Why do we think of iodine as that little bottle with skull and cross bones in the medicine cabinet? When did iodine information disappear from medical schools and medical libraries? Why?

Who stole iodine?

Iodine-based Medicine Time Line

15,000 BC	Monte Verde archaeological site reveals "medical hut" with seaweed medicines.
2,700 BCE	Chinese *Pen Tao* famous herbal pharmacopoeia documents seaweed for goiter and tumors.
1550 BCE	Eber's Papyrus Egyptian Medical Documents use of seaweed for breast cancer.
460 BC	Hippocrates, the founder of Modern Medicine recommends seaweed for goiter.
100 AD	Pliny the Elder, naturalist, lawyer, philosopher, promotes using burnt seaweed for goiter.
400 AD	Seaweeds used by Chinese physician Ke-Hung for goiter.
Middle ages	Avicenna and Galen, philosopher-doctors, recommend seaweed.
1779	UK, The Coventry Remedy published burned "spunge" profitable secret formula.
1811	Bernard Courtois discovers the new element Iodine while making gun powder from burned seaweed.
1813	New element confirmed by Humphry Davy and announced after wrangling among competing scientists in UK and Europe about who "discovered" the significance of the discovery.

| 1813 | New element officially named "Iode" by JL Lussac for the violet color of the vapor. |

1815–1816   First claimed use of iodine for goiter by William Prout, MD.

1819   Coindet officially introduces to practice, Tincture of Iodine as a specific for goiter, claiming it can reduce goiter in one week (validated 75 years later).

1820s   Inhalation of iodine vapors is practiced for lung ailments (seaweeds formerly scattered around hospital rooms). Many publications follow, as lung disease was prevalent in Europe. Iodine inhalation devices and inhalation lockets appeared.

1821   As part of the new French pharmacy movement, Francois Magendie added Iodine to a pharmacopoeia. Physicians tried it on every conceivable condition: croup, asthma, gangrene, gout, deafness, ulcers, to name just a few.

1829   Physician Jean Lugol invents Lugol's solution for tuberculosis, the scourge of Europe. Lugol's finds broader application as the preferred treatment. Revived in 2005 to the present.

1830   Sir Charles Sycamore publishes *Cases illustrating the Remedial Power of the Inhalation of Iodine and Conium in Tubercular Phthisis.*

1830s	Most widely used for tertiary syphilis. Brain surgery considered malpractice without a trial of iodine first since syphilitic lesions may resolve with iodine. Syphilitic Vincent Van Gogh writes his brother Theo, "You gotta try this stuff. It really helps." (Translation from French by the author.)
1831	JB Boussingalt suggests iodizing salt to prevent goiter. (It would take 100 years to accomplish that.)
1831–18??	The concept of iodine deficiency is proposed.
1840s	Dr. Jean Velpeau and others publish case studies on iodine in breast and ovarian disease.
1840s	Iodine used topically on breasts to diminish breast pain.
1851	The Great Exhibition at the Crystal Palace in Hyde Park exhibited many iodine compounds by ten pharmaceutical firms.
1860s	Civil War battlefield legend; iodine canteens carried.
	Iodine held as a field hospital staple as well as in soldier first aid kits in World Wars I and II plus the Vietnam war. Iodine, gauze and safety pins survived multiple incarnations as battlefield medicine.

1862	First record of tincture of iodine used as a battlefield antiseptic. Large amounts carried in canteens.
1864	The First British Pharmacopoeia publishes a selection of 14 preparations.
	Iodine documented as administered in baths, tablets, drops, topical application, injection, ionization and electrophoresis, soaps, salves, syrups, wines, powders, suppositories, and as a vapor.
1883	Publication: Iodine injected into sebaceous cysts successfully cures.
1899	Merck Manual: Iodine is the most used substance for tumors.
1899	Iodine suppositories manufactured for prostate disease and hemorrhoids.
1900	Iodine salves widely used for breast and other pain.
1910	Iodine-embedded lockets designed to prevent germ inhalation are distributed by the British Red Cross.
1913–1930	EC Kendall of Mayo shows the thyroid is 65 percent iodine.
1924	Michigan, USA: David Marine gets salt iodized after experiments in Michigan show school children developed less goiter when

taking iodine. US Army orders smaller-necked shirts because goiter incidence drops after salt iodization.

1930s   South Carolina discovers its iodine rich soil; declares itself "The Iodine State" on car license plates. Moonshiners take up the state spirit, coining the slogan, "Not a Goiter in a Gallon."

1948–1961   Articles published on rats by Jan Wolff and Israel Chaikoff, postulating iodine harmful to the thyroid. Although unverified, the information influences three generations of medical students.

1956   The International Index publishes 1700 approved pharmaceutical and proprietary names for iodine.

1961   Francis C. Kelley addresses the Royal Society of Medicine, lamenting the passing of Iodine out of fashion:

And what of the future? Who can tell how the reputations of iodine today will stand 100 years hence? To venture an opinion based on the events of the past, I can only say that the process of research, reevaluation, reappraisal, refinement will go on, and that in the year 2061 some iodine merits that enjoy contemporary favor will plainly appear ephemeral, while new merits as yet hidden from us will assuredly have declared themselves.

We may safely leave it to our successors to share the surprises that time has yet in store.

2000   F. Guy Abraham, MD, initiates a research project on iodine deficiency, reviewing the history of iodine research.

2005   "The Wolff-Chaikoff Effect: Crying Wolf?" by Guy E. Abraham, MD, is published.

2005   Jorge Flechas, MD, speaks at the Cancer Control Convention, LA, on Iodine, distributes Dr. Abraham's work.

2005   September, Lynne Farrow reports on Dr. Flechas' talk and Dr. Abraham's writings to cancer groups and begins researching for Breast Cancer Choices Iodine Investigation Project.

2006   January, Zoe Alexander creates Yahoo Iodine Group.

2006   March, Zoe creates *Iodine4Health.com* website to establish a repository for iodine research. The website has been reconstructed as *IodineResearch.com*

2006   October, Laura Olsson, Steve "Trapper" Wilson and Chris E. Vulcanel founded the Curezone Iodine Forum.

2006-7   Iodine Questions and Answers assembled and curated by Curezone Iodine Forum.

2006	November, Dr. Brownstein presents "Iodine: The Most Misunderstood Nutrient" at ACAM.
2006	Dr. Brownstein publishes *Iodine: Why You Need It, Why You Can't Live Without It.*
2007	February, First Iodine Conference (Scottsdale). Dr. Shevin's Salt Loading Protocol published on *BreastCancerChoices.org.*
2007	*Breast Cancer Choices* publishes The Iodine Protocol as recommended by the Iodine Conference.
2007	October, Second Iodine Conference (San Diego).
2007	Breast Cancer Choices creates Iodine Investigation Project measuring urinary iodine levels in breast cancer patients.
2007	Additional online groups and websites begin to explore iodine deficiency.
2007–Present	Iodine discussed on radio, television, videos and in additional conferences.
2012	*www.IodineResearch.com* founded as the Resource Network for the Iodine Movement. Mission: compiling research materials documenting the legacy of the Iodine Movement as well as peer review studies. The website was established to build on the work of Zoe Alexander's former website, *Iodine4Health.com.*

More Iodine Stories

Meet Virginia: Read her description of years of misery gradually improving.

I have been reading the Iodine Forum since the end of last year. The information that I found here has helped me so much! I learned a lot by reading how people reacted to taking <u>iodine</u> and how they dealt with the detox. Thank you all so much! So, here's my story.

I have been hypothyroid since I was 24. It started really slowly: just tiredness at first. After five years or so, I started to become emotionally unstable. I was paranoid, frightened, scared and unhappy. A friend said to me: "You're always tired." And I was. Still, I didn't really realize how much more tired I was than any healthy person should be. The decline was so gradual.

I got worse and worse ... I was in a lot of pain. Everything hurt. My joints, my muscles, my insides, everything. And I was always sooo tired. I didn't want to do anything. Not go to birthdays, no walks, no nothing.

Symptoms:

Allergies (hay fever, mites allergy, cannot tolerate perfume, suspected Hashimoto's); bad candida infection (vagina, gut and mouth); menstrual pains (uterus, lower back radiating to whole back and shoulders and neck); outer eyebrows gone; burn easily in the sun, hearing is bad especially in groups; tinnitus; bad memory (short term and long term): I cannot leave a pan on the stove and go do something else: it burns; tremors in eye lid; slow thinking: I could not follow a conversation/movie/book; cannot concentrate; underside of <u>feet</u> hurt; all joints feel like they are burning; gut hurt (even worse when pressed); the slightest physical exercise or house work results in rapid heartbeat, profuse sweating, red face, muscle pain and inflamed tendons; ganglion on back of hand; pain in left knee (other than the burning sensation); nose and throat tonsils and lungs inflamed at a regular basis (once a month); weight gain (my heaviest was 95 kilos); cannot tolerate carbs (not even full grain, not even beans); out of breath after taking three steps on the stairs; cold sore on lower lip (has been so big as to reach my jawbone); depression. During that period, I went to a doctor a few times. He told me to just take it more slowly.

At the age of 34, I weighed 95 kilos [209 pounds], was always tired, was bloated, in pain all the time, couldn't tolerate any carbs (by then I was on Atkins because carbs made my heart race and made me feel as if I would die), couldn't think straight, was unreasonable and had dark clouds in my head (that's what the depression felt like).

I again went to a doctor (I had just moved, so it was a different one this time). He again told me to take it easy. I replied that, if I took it any more easy than I was doing now, I might as well go and lay in my coffin right away. I started to cry out of frustration (first time I did that; I never cried). Probably to get rid of me he "allowed" me to have my blood tested. When the results came back, it was clear that I was hypothyroid. I was so relieved that they found something (little did I know).

At the age of 34, I was placed on thyroid hormone, T4 only. This doctor knew very little about thyroid illnesses and put me on a high dose immediately. I felt extremely ill from that: I couldn't walk a mile. Any exertion would make me breathless, and in extreme pain. At that point, I could not work anymore. My boss at the time was very understanding (until then, I hadn't called in sick very often, I simply went to bed straight out of work). I couldn't work for a whole year. I just lay on the couch or in bed and felt miserable.

After a year, I felt about as bad as I did before I started the T4. I started working again. Still had to get to bed as soon as I got home. I read a lot about Hypo-T and decided I wanted to try the desiccated form of thyroid meds. My doctor said that those kinds of meds were too unreliable. So then I asked to be allowed to take T3 instead (alongside the T4). He thought that was nonsense too. But this time I was determined and I asked to be sent to a specialist (in Holland you have to have a referral). I had researched to which doctor I wanted to go, and he relented. The specialist thought T3 was nonsense too, but gave it to me anyway.

The T3 gave me back my capacity to think. It also made me feel less cold. The first time I took T3, some kind of electric pulse shot to my toes, fingers and head. It helped a lot. The other symptoms remained though ...

Through the years I had to up my T4 from 100 mcg to 137 mcg. My TSH was no longer measurable. Doc said I was hyper. I disagreed and said I was hypo. I still had the classic signs of hypo (cold, ...) and none of the hyper.

My list of symptoms was still the same and I got progressively worse. I would get ill every month. It always started with my nose tonsils, then the throat tonsils, and then my lungs. I would be rid of it only one week in the month. It exhausted me. I also still had the tiredness, the pain in my joints, the fog in my brain (better after T3, but not resolved. I had to be in bed by 20:00 and sleep to 06:30 to not get sick and have a little energy.

I always kept reading a lot about hypo-T, hoping to find something I could do myself. And to be honest: to get out of the grip of my GP, who was trying to get me to lower my T4.

I discovered I had mercury poisoning when someone suggested mercury could be a problem. I started taking selenium for that. Selenium made me feel happier and think more clearly.

Reading about mercury poisoning led me to iodine. I started taking kelp, but it didn't do much for me. Then I found Curezone in October, 2011.

In November, 2011, I started on Lugol's Iodine. I took 50 mg twice a day. I got hyper, and I lowered my T4 dose accordingly. The effect was temporary though, and I upped to the original dose again (back to 137 mcg). This was such a disappointment! Then I read Dr. Brownstein's book where he said that it might take up to three years to see any significant improvement in the thyroid. So I had to be patient (which I am not)). I also started to gain weight.

My candida really hated the Lugol's (and because of that I loved it). I also took the companion supplements.

After reading a lot on Curezone, I decided to up my iodine by taking SKII. Now I took 100 mg of Lugol's and 50 mg of SKII. Again I got hyper, lowered my T4. This time I didn't need to up it back! I was now on 125 mcg/day T4. I also still take my T3. I don't lower that, it has a half-time of a day, whereas the T4 has a half-time of a week.

28th Feb 2012: I am now on 150 mg Lugol's and 300 mg SKII daily. A lot is happening to my body:

Spots on my hands are disappearing. My allergies are gone. Pain in left knee is about half as bad as it used to be. Losing weight, but more than that: my body is starting to look different. Face is not puffy anymore. My muscle strength is coming back. I'm soooo much happier! My head is wonderfully clear. My feet do not hurt anymore. Heart rate has gone down (except when I'm hyper, of course). I love going on a visit now. I have much more energy, and when I get tired, I just sit down for 15 minutes, and then I'm ready to go again. When hypo-T, resting didn't make any difference. Joints don't burn anymore. Tonsillitis is much better, but not resolved. I walked up a hill last week with my husband, and I could keep up with him without even panting or my heart racing!

Remaining symptoms:

Menstrual pains (just read here that might be a B12 deficiency. I just ordered the Dr. Brownstein's B 12 book). I get horrible pains in my lower back and shoulders. These pains stay for about a week after the bleeding has stopped. I still have intermittent bleeding too. I think my candida is almost under control. I still get the rapid heartbeats sometimes and still cannot tolerate carbs. Short term memory still bad. Gut still hurts. Diarrhea often.

So, a lot is better, but I'm not there yet. But then, I've been ill for more than 15 years now, and I've only been on Iodine for four months! The improvement is amazing!

Chapter Sixteen

Who Stole Iodine from My Medicine?

The beginning of wisdom is found in doubting; by doubting we come to the question, by seeking we may come upon the truth.

—Pierre Abelard, French philosopher

After World War II, the invention of penicillin and sulfa drugs began to replace iodine for infections. But the invention of antibiotics doesn't explain why a century of non-infection uses of iodine gradually lost favor, as if all the old books and articles were buried. My late mother-in-law's jar of Iodex Ointment was no longer available at Walgreens. Doctors began to know iodine only as a surgical antiseptic or an ingredient in radioactive contrast dyes. Most non-doctors of my generation only remember iodine as that little brown bottle in the medicine chest emblazoned with a skull and cross bones.

Where did the wealth of iodine information from the medical books and monographs go? Why did it disappear?

Remember, we are talking about a huge list of conditions from prostatitus to goiter to allergies. Iodine couldn't suddenly stop working after a hundred years. Some other forces must have contributed to the disappearance of iodine information. How could Iodine go from being used for dozens of medical conditions to being considered a poison? How could this happen? What turned the world against iodine?

Who stole iodine? In 2005, Guy Abraham, MD, wrote an article that answered that question. *The Wolff-Chaikoff Effect: Crying Wolff*, identified an influential paper published in 1948 which persuaded physicians that iodine was dangerous and would stop the thyroids of iodine-takers from working.

Dr. Abraham points out that the authors made a mistake by claiming iodine caused goiter in rats at 20 times the recommended daily allowance (RDA). *They, in fact, had not even bothered to check the rats' thyroid hormone level and reported no evidence of enlarged thyroid or disease.*

The Wolff-Chaikoff Assumption

This mistaken conclusion was repeated by Wolff again in 1969 when another paper extrapolated the findings to humans. Meanwhile one of the authors, Dr. Wolff, moved from U C Berkeley to the National Institutes of Health, inflating the importance of the study. The influence of Wolff-Chaikoff conclusions were so wide, the phenomenon was institutionalized by calling the fear-mongering event, "The Wolff-Chaikoff Effect." Medical textbooks perpetuated this mistake and taught it to at least three generations of doctors.

No one ever fact-checked or replicated the study, so its warning to avoid iodine supplementation was incorporated into medical practice.

A moratorium on human iodine research ensued. I'd read about the legendary Wolff-Chaikoff Effect in sources from textbooks to Wikipedia. But I had never personally heard anyone invoke Wolff-Chaikoff as a prophecy of doom that iodine would make them terribly sick.

Then at 8 o'clock one March morning, my phone rang. It was a Connecticut doctor saying that a patient who was in our Iodine Investigative Project database was sitting in his office. Her TSH (thyroid stimulating hormone) was out of the laboratory range, and he was terrified she had become desperately hypothyroid from taking iodine. He shared:

> Barbara has always had an intuitive sense of what works for her, which is why I'm calling you before taking her off iodine.

I asked if she had any other indications of being hypothyroid and he said, "No, she never looked or felt better."

In answering, I paraphrased a paper written by Dr. Jorge Flechas on why TSH levels may appear abnormal on iodine supplementation, but those anomalies are unlikely to reflect hypothyroidism.

> "Miss Farrow, it is a fundamental law of physiology that iodine shuts down the thyroid."

I let the words settle in my ears because I had never heard the disastrous Wolff-Chaikoff Effect legacy articulated so bluntly.

I referred him to Dr. Abraham's article on Wolff-Chaikoff and said I would fax him Dr. Flechas' paper explaining the TSH levels. As an afterthought, I added, "Would you please email me back to let me know your thoughts?" He agreed. A month later, he emailed me thanking me for the heads up on Wolff-Chaikoff,

TSH levels and the introduction to Dr. Abraham's online Iodine Project library.

Hearing the chilling pronouncement from a doctor so well-meaning that he would call a non-doctor for information made an impression on me. The disastrous legacy of Wolff-Chaikoff wasn't buried in a medical library anymore. It was alive and well in Connecticut and probably everywhere else. The notion that "iodine shuts down the thyroid gland" was still enforced as a "fundamental law of physiology" and still actively practiced. *Except that it turned out to be wrong—neither fundamental nor a law.* Just an assumption from an influence-leader with credentials from UC Berkeley and the National Institutes of Health. The "They must know what they're doing" mindset prevailed and soon there was a moratorium on further iodine research on humans. Sound crazy? Yes, but very true!

If iodine could be stolen from needy patients for decades by two unverified scientific papers, we must blame a medical system that allows unverified studies to determine patient care.

Yes, that's an accusation. How could this fiasco happen? Isn't anybody paying attention? How many people have been harmed by the theft of iodine from medical practice? Me? You? Our children?

The most important scientific revolutions all include, as their only common feature, the dethronement of human arrogance from one pedestal after of previous conviction about the centrality in the cosmos.

—Stephen Jay Gould

The Abraham Challenge Creates a Revolution

Dr. Abraham, a former Professor of Obstetrics, Gynecology, and Endocrinology at the UCLA School of Medicine, did not keep his findings to himself. He continued to publish more on iodine deficiency and enlisted the partnership of two extraordinary physicians in clinical practice, Jorge Flechas, MD, of North Carolina, and David Brownstein, MD, of Michigan. Since 2005, the three passionate, committed doctors produced a body of work that has created a revolution in existing assumptions about iodine.

Why? Because their work has been tested as tried and true by an inestimable number of patients and doctors over the last seven years.

If this information had come out 20 years ago, the revolution in iodine thinking would not have occurred. There was no Internet 20 years ago. No sophisticated patient-to-patient network. No rapid communications between physicians.

The Iodine Doctors' claims about the benefits of iodine supplementation could have remained an issue quietly discussed at medical conferences. Best case, iodine might have been used by a small group of thinking doctors for its most popular benefits, or it could have just faded without a trace. The resulting patient outcome may have been of high quality but limited by:

- The few iodine literate doctors; and
- The fact that these doctors could be open to criticism and thus would treat conservatively in dosing iodine. The true benefits of iodine could have languished for another twenty years.

But the Iodine doctors went out into the medical community and spoke about iodine deficiency at conferences. They cited case after case from breast disease to insulin reduction to depression. Patient activists attending these events reported back to their online communities. They enlisted their peers to help them investigate. They read all of Dr. Abraham's articles and checked his citations. They listened to Dr. Flechas' radio interviews. They read Dr. Brownstein's book. The communities like Breast Cancer Choices set out to investigate the information by researching iodine's historical benefits as well as the mysterious politics of iodine-based medicine.

These communities set out to determine the validity of iodine usage: Was it safe? If it was, what diseases and conditions could be benefited by it? Or, was it unsafe? Was there a supplement that was readily available that could do widespread good right under our noses. What were the facts? What was the fiction?

The Iodine Revolution contains two inter-dependent parts, the original thinker and the grass roots movement which proved Dr. Abraham right.

As online participants are mostly anonymous, challenges to the pro-iodine information came fast, encouraging competition to get at the facts. By 2006, the first online groups sprang up with the exclusive purpose of investigating iodine. Zoe, a former psychology professor, established The Yahoo Iodine Group which was later moderated by others. The Curezone Iodine Forum, created by Steve Wilson, Laura Olsson and Chris E. Vulcanel, started almost simultaneously. Their memberships caught fire as good results and excitement grew. Predictably, several Internet pundits predicted all the iodine-takers would be dead in six months from the legendary and widely held/practiced belief in the Wolff-Chaikoff Effect.

But the pro-iodine participants continued experimenting, supporting each other and collecting testimonials. Some pro-iodine-thought leaders had medical or science backgrounds, so they weighed the evidence in the iodine medical literature. Laura Olsson became a tireless historian-anthropologist of iodine's use. Her blog records much valuable information that would be lost to history without her research. See: *http://iodinehistory.blogspot. com.* Excitement grew as new information was rapidly shared and rechecked. Clearly, Wolff-Chaikoff would never have gotten past these patient-to-patient Internet investigators.

Solidarity and respect grew between the various online forums and webmasters as we all learned from each other. Doctors in clinical practice began to learn from the patients' information exchange. Breast Cancer Choices kept track of many of the informed Iodine Practitioners and compiled their contact information in an international *Iodine Literate Practitioners Directory.*

The Iodine Revolution: The Iodine Movement Steals Back Iodine from Obscurity

An apparently arbitrary element, compounded of personal or historical accident, is always a formative ingredient of the beliefs espoused by a given scientific community at a given time."
—T. S. Kuhn, The Structure of Scientific Revolutions

In 1980, more patients were more likely to follow the status quo because medical information was monopolized by credentialed practitioners and access to medical information was limited. By 2005, the Internet had overthrown the monopoly on medical information via a variety of resources, starting with the references at *Pubmed.com,* the online database of the National Library of Medicine, which became available to all.

Within a couple of years, Google digitized old medical books scanned from libraries around the world, creating a bounty for research. Old newspapers and magazines were now searchable. Such resources fueled brainstorming by patient-to-patient groups and transformed what we know about medicine.

Pre-Internet, it might have taken 20 or 30 years to reverse an accepted medical idea. Now the Internet has shown that a savvy patient-to-patient network can create a revolution in medical thinking much, much faster.

In 1980, the overwhelming number of patient-activists did not exist to fact-check and experiment. The numbers not only enabled evidence gathering, the numbers of iodine users grew loud, credible and capable of spreading the message.

When the Iodine Movement first gained traction on *www. breastcancerchoices.org*, Karen, one of our Breast Cancer Think Tank members, asked, "If iodine is so good, why doesn't the Life Extension Foundation sell it?" I remember answering, "It's just a matter of time." And, of course, that prediction proved true. Lugol's and Iodoral are now available everywhere due to customer demand.

The Iodine Revolution: The Grass Roots Steals Back Iodine

When we describe Dr. Abraham's challenge to prevailing myths about iodine as revolutionary, is that just hype?

According to T.S. Kuhn, the author of *The Structure of Scientific Revolutions*, the word, "revolution" refers to a shift in power due to a shift in thinking. Thinking differently translates into shifting entrenched assumptions to an opposite perspective. An opposite perspective translates into opposite actions.

**The so-called fundamental law of physiology—
that iodine can shut down the thyroid gland—has
been challenged, overthrown and even reversed.**

Dr. Abraham was the original thinker who looked at Wolff-Chaikoff Effect studies and didn't observe the same phenomena or reasoning which had made its way into textbooks. He looked at the history of iodine and saw the Wolff-Chaikoff characterization as a brief interval in medical history wrong-headedness that caught on. As Kuhn says, history is not usually taken seriously by doctors. They put their faith in the present, not the past. Doctors usually see knowledge as evolving, not devolving.

The power of a runaway bad idea can be unstoppable for generations until someone questions it, and this is what happened; because Dr. Abraham not only discovered the bad idea, *he set out to unmask it*. He stopped the runaway bad idea. Doctors, such as Dr. David Derry in Canada who wrote *Iodine and Breast Cancer*, and Dr. Jonathan Wright, who had been using potassium iodide in his practice, supported Abraham's mission. They were pro-iodine but did not systematically decide to challenge the authority of the Wolff-Chaikoff thinking as Dr. Abraham had.

Historical Importance of the Wolff-Chaikoff Reversal

The Iodine Movement created a revolution in thinking, not just because Dr. Abraham created a shift in thinking about iodine, but because he created a *reversal in thinking*. Iodine has been *redefined* from a poison to a vital nutrient with life-changing benefits. From a dusty bottle in the back of the medicine cabinet bearing a skull and cross bones to a supplement health food stores can't keep on the shelves.

The Iodine Movement has applied Dr. Abraham's research and found new ways to revive the rich history of a 15,000-year-old iodine medicine. We have stolen back the iodine information. The tens of thousands of people in the Iodine Movement are a walking refutation of Wolff-Chaikoff.

"Historians must recapture the past and work the present," writes T.S. Kuhn. But reverse engineering in medicine is laughed at. The premise persists that if an idea is new, it must be right. When Dr. Abraham documented that the 150 years of iodine use had proved safe, his report challenged the medical industry dictum that anything new must be better. Iodine's long history provided momentum for Iodine Movement activists. The more history was unearthed, the more compelling was the rationale for iodine.

To this day, whenever I speak on iodine, the audience tells me the most memorable information is the historical use of iodine. They remember the Civil War iodine canteen I hold up and the iodine locket I show that was used during Influenza epidemics by The British Red Cross. They remember Van Gogh writing his brother about how iodine helped his syphilis. They remember the hundred and forty year-old, yellowed letter from the woman writing to her sister about how iodine helped her breast pain.

Wolff-Chaikoff created an Iodine Prohibition Movement completely contrary to a century of evidence which produced volumes of books supporting iodine as beneficial and even miraculous.

How could Wolff-Chaikoff create such a change in the laws of physiology in the face of this contradiction? How many women and men have suffered, yes, even died, because Wolff-Chaikoff's conclusions that became the law of medicine? Should we care now that the truth has been exposed?

The answer is an emphatic, "We must!"

We should care how this happened because other such wrong-headed ideas might dominate other treatment regimens where the stakes are high. Wolff-Chaikoff Effect thinking has lasted five decades and is on its way out, but probably has several years left until the final straggler reviews the evidence and clinical reports.

History will reflect that the Wolff-Chaikoff Effect has been transformed into the Wolff-Chaikoff *Interval,* a period of time when a flawed theory made its way into medical practice and research because of lack of peer diligence. A lack of peer diligence that has harmed untold numbers.

Thoughts

- What other flawed thinking is out there in the medical textbooks, totally accepted and totally wrong? How long will it take to change thinking? Who is brave enough to challenge the text books and withstand the scoffing?

- Changes in thinking equals changes in action equals changes in relationships equals shifts in power relationships. The debunking of the Wolff-Chaikoff thinking can provide a gateway event to the challenge of other authoritarian notions. That is, if medical consensus got that wrong, what else did they get wrong? How many have been harmed or died from it?

- The fall of the Wolff-Chaikoff Interval provides a great learning experience to those who possess the courage to believe their own observations and reasoning rather than what has been handed down as law.

More Iodine Stories

Meet Don: Fibromyalgia results lead to Lugol's application to testicles.

I have been taking Iodine orally for several years because of fibromyalgia pain. It really worked although it took me a while to get up to the 50 mg because I was resistant to taking the salt water. Then I found if you put the sea salt into gelatin capsules, you don't have to actually drink salt water.

Then I recently heard of the topical painting of Lugol's solution directly on the testicles so I thought I'd give it a try. I tried one drop at a time mixed with Laura's Organics iodine salve. Only when I got up to 15 drops did I feel something odd in my genitals. My organs seemed to wake up. I hope researchers will explore this. Women have publicized the benefits of iodine for female problems but men have hung back. I wish more guys would try this and report their results.

Meet Joan: Pomphlyx eczema resolves.

I'm taking Iodine to prevent a recurrence of breast cancer. I had many observations when I initially took iodine, most of which I have forgotten.

However, one complaint I have had diagnosed is a kind of eczema known as pomphlyx here in the UK. If I don't take a MINIMUM of 2 drops Lugol's Iodine most days, my eczema starts to develop on my fingers and feet. It always goes when I resume iodine. I started high dose MSM recently (one of my experimental forays!) and the eczema came back quite aggressively. I increased my iodine and got the balance right, and away it went.

My nephew also controls his eczema now with iodine.

Meet Melinda: Sinus and allergy issues resolve with money saving alternative.

I started 50 mg Iodoral when Stephanie B mentioned it after I was diagnosed with thyroid cancer. My use was scattered, depending on my finances. After breast cancer, I upped it to 200 mg.

I have had sinus issues forever, usually with one or two sinus infections in the spring and again in the fall. I have many allergies. An early season like this one would have normally caused me a lot of misery, but I've sailed through it this year. I am back to 100 mg now due to finances. I use to spend approximately $42 monthly on DeHist, a natural antihistamine to keep sinuses from bothering me.

Meet Alice: Breast calcifications, coldness, hair loss, Raynaud's Disease, all clearing up or resolved.

I started using iodine about 18 months ago when I decided not to get a stereotactic biopsy for suspicious calcifications. I took an iodine loading test. I was only slightly deficient, about 15 percent but the doctor advised me to take 100 mg daily of Iodoral along with ATP cofactors in case of an early stage of cancer.

About six months ago I had an ultrasound of the area and, after careful examination, there were no visible calcifications. I did not get a mammogram as I do not want to have one anymore, but I knew that the calcifications picked up on my last mammogram had also been seen on the ultra sound. Also, thermographs showed improvement and less inflammation in the area.

Iodine has done wonders for me. Fibrocystic disease is clearing up. I also think that I may have had a sluggish thyroid that was not picked up on blood tests as now my feet are no longer cold, my Raynaud's Disease has gone away and my alopecia (hair loss) is almost resolved.

Now I am taking 50 mg of Iodoral a day as it will probably take another few years, to totally resolve fibrocystic disease.

I took other measures that I researched but I think the Iodoral was the main player in my success. I hope my story helps others.

Thanks to people like you for the work you do.

Chapter Seventeen

Who Stole Iodine From My Food?

*We know from world studies that if you give iodine
during pregnancy the babies that come out are usually
20-30 points higher in IQ than their parents.*

—Jorge Flechas, MD, MPH

**Figure 8
Table 1 from the National Center
for Health Statistics**

Iodized Salt Consumption Drops 50%

National Center for Health Statistics ... Monitoring the Nation's Health

NHANES 1 1971–74	NHANES II 2000
32.00	16.1

163

The National Center for Health Statistics, the government agency that measures nutrients, reported that people tested in 2000 excreted *half* the iodine in their urine than those tested in 1971–1974.

After 1972, Iodine Gone from Bread!

Researchers believe the drop in urinary iodine levels comes from when iodine was removed from bread and baked goods around 1970.

In the 1960s, the average slice of bread contained 150 mcg iodine in the form of potassium iodate. Even one slice contained the RDA (recommended daily allowance). Public health officials and food scientists regard iodine as a fortificant, a substance that provides nutrients that are easy to miss in adequate quantities without adding them to common foods. When iodine in the form of potassium iodate was added to bread, the average person might consume several slices of bread a day through sandwiches, breakfast toast or other baked goods, so the average iodine consumption was at least a milligram per day. That was a significant amount to protect the thyroid. Also, iodate in bread is absorbed very efficiently and made an excellent dough conditioner.

We're waiting for a researcher to access bread companies' files and see if we can trace back why iodine was removed across the board from most commercial breads. Did some official feel iodine was harmful in the wake of the Wolff-Chaikoff era?

A 1970 conference report from the Food and Nutrition Board, National Academy of Sciences, titled *Iodine Nutriture in the United States,* strongly hints that iodine in bread may not be safe and that iodized salt is superior. The scientists also report that it is difficult to get a readable radioactive-iodine medical scan since the population became more iodine sufficient. The uptake of the scanning chemicals could not penetrate tissues that were iodine replete. So the radioactive scans only lit up when people were iodine deficient? Were they suggesting public health policy should change, that people lower their iodine intake in order to get better radioactive iodine images? Does the importance of creating better images transcend the importance of iodine sufficiency? It looks that way.

The function of the report appears to be to raise insidious questions disguised as public concern—*Is iodate in bread dangerous?*

The report answers its own question by urging that iodized salt remain the Gold Standard. By 1980, wild claims were published. The USDA reports in *The Fortification of Foods: A Review*, that iodine as a disinfectant "has long been known to be *lethal* ..." [author's italics] and that Americans get more than enough iodine from non-bread sources, so [iodine] "should be replaced whenever possible by compounds containing less or no iodine."

Lethal? Any documentation of "lethal?" No.

No matter. Bye-bye iodine in bread. The bakery companies may have feared being sued if someone blamed their breads for a sickness after two public groups had scorned iodine as dangerous. Going along is always easier than bucking influence-leaders or checking facts.

What could be worse than removing the major source of dietary iodine? ... Putting the *anti-iodine* potassium bromate into commercial bread and flour. This policy change took effect in the early 1970s. How does bromine steal iodine? Bromine and iodine compete for the same receptors, so when bromate was added to replace iodate, dietary iodine from other sources sitting on those receptors was displaced. Bromate had been used earlier as a dough conditioner but was not brought in to replace iodine significantly until the anti-iodine sentiments began. *Was the removal of iodine from the food supply a down-stream result of the Wolff-Chaikoff thinking?*

What about the addition of bromate? That decision by the bakers appears to be accidental since bromate was already known as an effective dough conditioner comparable to iodine in creating pleasing bread. The bakers couldn't have foreseen the consequences ahead when additional bromines from fire retardants affected the toxic bromine load in human beings.

The Iodized Salt Scam

Whenever someone learns I'm writing about iodine, their eyes often glaze over because they assume there's really nothing to know about iodine. Recently, on a four-hour train ride between Boston and New York, I found myself sitting next to a well-groomed man reading the Wall Street Journal. His duffel had Clifford stamped on the side, and he talked to someone named Buffy on his cell phone every fifteen minutes. As I kept my head down, taking notes, he asked me what I was writing. "A book on iodine," I said.

"Oh, I know all about that. I use iodized salt all the time, though Buffy prefers the Himalayan pink salt." I find it hard to restrain myself in these cases. The diplomatic half of me wants to let the topic pass. The activist half of me wants to scream, "Iodized salt? You want to know about iodized salt? Don't get me started on iodized salt." The diplomatic half generally loses the battle and I stop everything to make my case against iodized salt. I can't help myself.

We have an iodine crisis in good part because of the iodized salt scam. It is the government recommendation that an adequate amount of iodine can be consumed from iodized salt.

So, how much iodine do you obtain and absorb from iodized salt? Anyone? Anyone?

No one really knows, because misleading information has created a three-part information scam. Whistle-blowers must challenge these government guidelines because they're based on inaccurate information and disproved assumptions that are harmful. The report, *Iodine Nutrition: Iodine Content of US Salt*, by Dasgupta, et al., discusses the "Iodine Gap." The gap refers to the amount of iodine that's supposed to be in iodized salt and what amount can actually be measured by the time you use it. The researchers also point out that salt is a poor food product to fortify because chloride, which is a halogen, competes with the iodine, making it less effective.

Scam 1. The average gram of iodized salt is thought to contain 0.075 mcg. But that measurement is taken at the factory. By the time the salt reaches the grocery store, half of the iodine in the sealed container has "vaporized," or as scientists would say, the salt "sublimed" into the air. Once you get the salt container to your kitchen and open it, whoosh, more iodine escapes. The longer you keep it, the less iodine remains. Iodine in salt is unstable. Dasgupta, et al., report it takes between 20 and 40 days for an opened container of iodized salt to lose half of its iodine. How long have you had that iodized salt in your pantry?

So when you factor in the loss of iodine into the air, the actual consumption of iodine through salt is completely theoretical. The amount the people add to the product is not what we actually get when we sprinkle iodized salt on our food. Do the math. The bottom line is, nobody knows how much iodine you get from iodized salt. There are too many variables. Was the salt warehoused? Do you live in a damp or warm area? How long has it been in your cupboard leaking iodine fumes into the universe?

Scam 2. But say you're an average man, standing outside the Morton factory and get the freshest, most iodized salt available. What are you getting? Even the most concentrated iodized salt is only 10 percent "bioavailable," meaning only a fraction gets absorbed. Iodide may be added to salt but remember, salt is sodium *chloride*. Chloride and iodide are both in the halogen family of elements so they compete with each other for the same receptors. Chloride has the ability to *cancel out* at least some of the benefit of iodide. Again, do the math. You're only absorbing 10 percent of whatever the good people at Morton put in the container. Unlike adding iodine to flour as potassium iodate, the iodine in salt is difficult to absorb. You certainly may get some iodine from iodized salt but what goes in doesn't necessarily get to the right places.

Scam 3. But say you're a *woman* standing outside the factory and get the freshest salt which is only 10 percent bioavailable, you're might get a protective amount, right? A protective amount if, say, *you consumed a pound a day?*

No. Not if you're a woman. The salt is iodized with potassium io*dide* which may be helpful to the thyroid. But the breasts and ovaries need io*dine* as well as io*dide*. This time, you can skip the math and just go straight to the science. Women are taking the wrong iodine.

Is there ever any reason to consume processed iodized salts in this time of Iodine Crisis? The answer is,

1. Only in an emergency when you need salt and can't access unprocessed salt.
2. Only if you can't afford iodine supplementation.

Taking iodized salt alone as a source of iodine actually only benefits communities too poor to get any other kind of iodine. Iodizing salt was meant to prevent goiter, but nothing else. The minimal iodized salt standard is, in fact, the "Goiter Standard," but does not reflect the needs of the other organs. The Goiter Standard of iodine provides a disappointingly low bar for the government to set when iodine helps prevent so many other illnesses. Skimping on the cheap cost of iodine means paying for more expensive problems down the line. Another thing to remember is that processed salts often come with controversial aluminum anti-caking chemicals. I wouldn't take aluminum-laced processed salt products unless I had a lot of cash socked away for future Alzheimer's care.

More Iodine Stories

Meet Marla: Lumpy, sore, fibrocystic breasts resolve. Energy improves.

I want to tell you about my experiences with Iodoral. It has been the most beneficial product I have ever used. I have fibrocystic breasts, which my gyno described as just lumpy, sore breasts. He said it really doesn't hurt you, it just hurts. Well, I think that is bull. I started doing some research on my own, ended up going to a chiro for a back problem. She had me lie on my stomach to adjust me, and, wow, did my breast hurt! Well, that was the best day of my "health" life! She did a manual lymphatic drainage and put me on Iodoral. The drainage relieved my pain immediately, but it came back within a day or so.

I continued with the Iodoral. My husband was the first one to notice a difference and link it to the Iodoral. In about three weeks, I just felt good. Really good. I had energy, I felt like going places and doing things. It was not a jittery caffeine energy; it was just what a normal 30-year-old should feel like. And my libido was back. That is what my husband noticed! Prior to the Iodoral, I just didn't want to be with my husband. I wanted to want to, but I just didn't. But suddenly, I wanted to!

And finally, on to my breast. My breast pain would start exactly 10 days before my period. And be very severe. On the second month, no pain before. None at all. And as long as I am on my Iodoral, it doesn't come back. If I am not on it, it comes back immediately. My mother had breast cancer at 38. I am now 35, I have taken control of my health, and I will not be a silent victim! Praise God for you and the work that you are doing for a cure! I believe that breast and thyroid cancer is just the beginning for Iodoral.

Meet Lydia's daughter: Hashimoto's Thyroiditis slowly improved antibodies.

My daughter has Hashi's. I then started her on Iodoral slowly building up to 150 mg. The antibody numbers kept coming down. I resisted starting her on Iodine at first because of the warnings I had heard about Hashi's and iodine. I was so nervous, but I'm so grateful we did it.

Meet Priscilla's dog, Abby: Cyst disappears.

My dog, Abby, has had a big lump or cyst on her back near her tail for a few years. The vet told me it was a sebaceous cyst and to leave it alone and try not to squeeze it (which I hadn't). A month ago after the appt. with the vet, I put some Lugol's Iodine on the area just to see what would happen. Last week I noticed that it seemed bigger and softer. Today I noticed that it had popped open and was draining on its own. I gently squeezed out the remaining pus and cleaned it with hydrogen peroxide and dabbed some more Lugol's on it. So the lump is gone, and she's doing great! Iodine is amazing stuff!

Chapter Eighteen

The Perfect Storm Theory of Breast Cancer

The absence of iodine in the human body is a promoter of cancer.

—Jorge Flechas, MD, MPH

You Call that *Normal*?

As a breast cancer survivor who has devoted a third of my life investigating how breast health can go terribly wrong, I found that experts snookered me many times. I believed what I was told. When my breasts felt tender or swollen, I was told that occasional pain and swelling were normal. This "normal" condition was so normal it had a name: "benign breast disease." I wasn't sure how a condition with benign as its first name and disease as its last name could still be called *normal*. When I raised this linguistic problem, I was told "benign breast disease is normal because it's so *common*."

Even a hundred years ago, when syphilis afflicted nearly 50 percent of the European population in the 1800s, nobody ever suggested it was normal.

> But if a disease is so common, wouldn't that
> make it an epidemic? Or some kind of massive public
> health problem? When did common equal normal?
> Fact-check my reasoning. A common-normal-
> benign-disease makes a double oxymoron, right?

Unfortunately, back then I was young and inexperienced, so when doctors gave me the double oxymoron explanation, I was not yet schooled enough to challenge authorities or assumptions. I surrendered my common sense to anybody carrying a clipboard or wearing a white coat. Assumption: *"They must know what they're doing."*

Only when I began my own independent research did I uncover the fact—the evidence—that benign breast disease can progress to cancer. I realized the extent of how badly I was misled with this normal-common-benign-breast disease myth. In fact, research shows breast cancer doesn't "strike," but most often develops slowly when the breasts are sick and inflamed. Not all sick breasts eventually develop cancer, but benign breast disease creates a high risk factor. Mayo Clinic research found that one third of women diagnosed with the benign breast disease, called atypical hyperplasia, will progress to invasive breast cancer within five years.

> What makes the breast, nature's most mysterious
> baby food factory, sick or inflamed? Since the
> condition is so common, you'd think scientists would
> be paying more attention or looking for a cause,
> asking why or identifying when, in the course of a
> woman's life, breast health starts to deteriorate.

Have you ever heard a doctor ask: "Why could you have sick breasts?" or "What have you been exposed to?" Medicine will ask, "How did you pick up that virus?" "Where have you been that you could have gotten that infection?" If you are diagnosed with mesothelioma, they will ask if you were exposed to certain carcinogens. Has anybody in the history of the universe been asked why their breasts are swollen, tender or lumpy? Show of hands. Anyone? Anyone?

Nobody.

At best, practitioners prescribe anti-inflammatory supplements such as evening primrose oil or Advil, or tell patients to avoid caffeine. But applying these "band aids" ignores the condition. If either of these strategies helps at all, they work by masking the underlying cause. Any inflammation may improve with anti-inflammatory meds, or less dehydrating caffeine. But what caused the inflammation in the first place? As Dr. David Brownstein would say,

Fibrocystic breast disease is not an Advil deficiency syndrome.

Our culture has been brainwashed with the myth that sick breasts are normal and that breast cancer strikes suddenly between mammograms; that one day your breasts appear perfectly healthy, and then, bang, some nasty white spot shows up on a mammogram. Scientists know breast cancers have been growing for seven or more years before detection but the pop culture myth of cancer striking instead of developing, persists. This erroneous message is marketed by the October *Breast Cancer Awareness Month*™ campaigns. Yes, you read that right. That's a trademark symbol after the name. Breast Cancer Awareness Month™ is trademarked by Astra-Zeneca, a drug company that manufactures breast cancer drugs. "Awareness" is a billion dollar industry.

But awareness of what? Cause? No. October might as well be renamed mammogram awareness month—all based on the breast cancer "strikes" myth. The Breast Cancer Industry is designed to manufacture bigger and better ways to close the barn door after the horse has bolted. The industry just wants to catch the horse, not fix the barn door.

The industry couldn't have picked a worse time to ignore preventable risk factors like benign breast disease. Pre-cancerous benign breast disease is a growing crisis. Dr. Jorge Flechas has reported that benign breast disease notations have increased on autopsy from 23 percent in 1928 to 89 percent in 1973. Not all benign disease progresses to full blown malignant disease, but many do. Mayo Clinic Oncologist Lynn Hartmann, M.D., has been studying the risk factors of benign breast disease progression. The *New England Journal of Medicine* reports that Hartmann and her team followed women with benign disease for 15 years to see how many developed breast cancer as compared to women without benign disease. Women diagnosed with "proliferative" benign disease were 88 percent more likely to develop breast cancer. Women with the more aggressive benign disease, atypical hyperplasia, were 4.2 times more likely to develop breast cancer than women with no history of benign disease.

So the dangers of benign disease are slowly getting publicity. Dr. Hartmann now serves as principal investigator for a Department of Defense Center of Excellence grant titled "Benign Breast Disease: Toward Molecular Prediction of Breast Cancer Risk."

But Medicine moves slowly. Most of us don't want to wait 15 years of our lives for research to tell us sick breasts are not normal. Breast cancer rates have risen from one in 20 in 1970 to one in eight by the year 2000. Younger and younger women are diagnosed with invasive breast cancer. How can young breasts be getting sick so fast? You would think that young breasts haven't been around long enough to get so sick. Given that it takes seven or more years for most breast cancer to be detectible, does it mean a palpable threat in the near future for 20-year-old women? Thirty-year-old women?

Figure 9
Increase in Breast Cancer Rates Since Iodine Was Removed from Flour and Bromate Was Added

Why Are Breast Cancer Rates Rising?

1968	2006
Lifetime Risk 1 in 20	Lifetime Risk 1 in 7-8

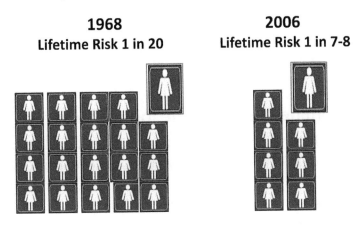

Breast cancer used to be a disease of aging women. No longer. Jennifer, a young operating room nurse, reports, "My breast pain has kept me from hugging anyone since I was twelve." Is she a future breast cancer victim?

What's going on? What could explain the rise in breast cancer? What other cancers are on the rise? Thyroid cancer has risen 182 percent since 1975. More women get thyroid cancer than men. Women require much more iodine to nourish the breasts and ovaries. Larger breasted women require even more iodine. Is there a Perfect Storm Theory of Thyroid Cancer also? Benign nodules and cysts also afflict these organs. What do the breasts, the ovaries and the thyroid have in common?

All three are dependent on iodine to develop and stay healthy with the ability to,

1. Receive nourishment, and
2. Clear out toxins.

Without an essential amount of iodine, the breasts and ovaries seem to get congested and swell. Cell membranes don't work. Without enough iodine, toxic fluids back up, causing enlargement and inflammation. Fluid collects in cysts. Ropey, fibrous tissue develops. Nodules may start growing. At its worst, fibrocystic breasts grow as hard as rocks. Nature's baby food factory behaves as if it's choking on a *poison*. Hmmm.

Bromine Poisoning the Iodine Receptors

Hold on. What if a specific, anti-iodine toxin actually does poison the breasts, ovaries and thyroids by purging the protective iodine from tissues? What if that *anti-iodine poison* is responsible for blocking tissues from receiving nourishment and circulating fluids? What if that poison was introduced into the environment in the 1970s as an element in flame retardants, pesticides and food additives? Could it be called the bromine family? Could the element bromine cause extreme iodine deficiencies by over-powering iodine at the cellular level. The answer is, *yes*.

The biochemists refer to such a process, where one element in the halide group dukes it out with another, as "competitive inhibition." When bromine dominates, iodine recedes. When bromine purges iodine, a deficiency results and the cells become poisoned and inflamed. The poison paradigm is just beginning to be explored with great encouragement because this form of poisoning is a reversible situation.

Figure 10
Bromide Dominance Leads to Iodine Deficiency

When stealth bromine exposure infiltrates the air, soil, cars, mattresses and more, what does this contamination do to Iodine?

When bromines dominate, iodine recedes from humans and animals.

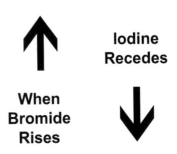

Iodine Recedes

When Bromide Rises

Nobody gets bromine poisoning overnight. It usually takes years for bromines to build up. Bromine fire retardants are technically characterized as "persistent toxins," meaning they don't metabolize out of the body as easily as other toxins might. Some bromines take up residence in the tissues and stay a very long time.

Figure 11
Perfect Storm Theory of Breast Cancer.

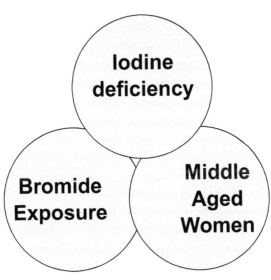

1970 The Perfect Storm Theory of Breast Cancer Begins

I developed the Perfect Storm Theory of Breast Cancer when I observed that bromide fire retardants and pesticides were introduced about the same time as iodate was replaced with bromate in bread. The rise in breast cancer corresponds with that time frame.

A Perfect Storm occurs when specific unrelated events come together at the same time to cause a disaster that might be insignificant if only one event occurred.

Event 1: Occurred in the 1970s when our major source of dietary iodine, the iodate form, used to fortify flour and baked goods, was **removed**. Event 1 was bad enough.

Event 2: Occurred when potassium *bromate,* a form of bromine, was **added**. Yes, an anti-iodine was added to replace iodine.

The second event makes the first event more catastrophic. What little dietary iodine might remain from eggs and ocean foods was now bullied from the body by the bromating of flour.

Event 3: But wait, there's more. The bromination of America didn't stop with flour. The Perfect Storm Theory of Breast Cancer identifies another major bromine invasion in the 1970s: the mass introduction of brominated fire retardants. Fire retardant chemical dust escapes from products like rugs, upholstery, stuffed animals, mattresses, cars and electronics we use every day.

We inhale the dust and it goes into our bloodstream and sequesters itself in the tissues, the endocrine system, the brain. Although fire retardant dust is the most grievous source of bromine; there are countless other sources that flow into our bodies from brominated vegetable oil (BVO) in certain sodas, sports drinks and foods. We are surrounded with bromine and bromides, an insidious element known to sedate, to suppress the thyroid, disrupt reproduction and even cause mental illness. Bromine fire retardants are even found in breast milk. Bromide is banned in many countries but not in the US. The question becomes: Why not here?

Then the fad of avoiding salt caught on along with the notion that iodine was a chemical additive. Check your supermarket. Only half of the available salt is iodized. Some people believe iodine is a chemical additive. Even if people do consume iodized salt, iodine in salt is not absorbed nearly as well as from flour. Iodized salt gives people a false sense of security. In 2000, The National Center for Health statistics found that people were consuming 50 percent less iodine than they had approximately 30 years before.

Subtracting iodine and adding bromine creates a devastating scenario whereby bromine dominates and iodine recedes. Bromine exposure reduces the amount of iodine available to protect and nourish the breasts. Fluids accumulate. Cysts develop to wall-off toxins. Hormone receptors disrupt. Breast disease worsens.

What cheap, uncomplicated element has been found to reverse benign breast disease within one day to three months?

Iodine.

We know this from medical studies. We know from the thousands of women who have used iodine and documented their stories. We know this from the hundreds of Iodine Literate Practitioners from their clinical reports. When integrative medicine expert, Michael Schachter, MD, gave his iodine presentation at the American College for the Advancement of Medicine Conference in 2010, he asked the audience how many of them were currently prescribing iodine to their patients. half of the practitioners raised their hands!

When I let people know I was writing a book on iodine and was looking for reports from iodine takers, I received so many emails from fibrocystic breast disease patients that I couldn't possibly use all the striking and heart-warming stories of improvement and healing of sometimes lifelong afflictions.

If iodine can drive out the toxin, there must be something about the antidote that is important to keeping the breasts healthy. This is where the Perfect Storm Theory of Breast Cancer comes in. It is the story of the poison and the antidote.

But **Event 4** of the perfect storm comes into play when baby boomers and post baby boomers begin to get into pre-menopausal states where their hormones become erratic and they need their hormone receptors and breast tissues to be functioning optimally, for the receptors to be clean and the tissues free from toxins. Middle aged women are most vulnerable to breast cancer and more likely to suffer from endocrine disruption from bromines.

The Perfect Storm Theory of Breast Cancer

Mechanism of Action?

Iodine has so many mechanisms of action that it's still unclear precisely how it works in every situation, including the breast. Dr. Guy Abraham reported that the term, "deobstruent" (drives out toxins), was used in the 1800s by physicians who observed the iodine "tamp down" of infection, swelling, skin, endocrine and other abnormalities. Since then, science has learned how essential iodine is for both the development and maintenance of healthy vital organs. But it's clear that , as one doctor phrased it, "the breasts love iodine." According to a study done by iodine pioneer Bernard Eskin, MD, way back in 1974, sick breasts absorbed twice as much radioactive iodine as normal breasts.

Figure 12
Abnormal Breasts Took Up
Twice As Much Radioactive Iodine

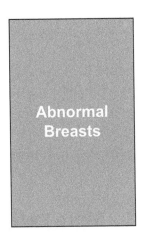

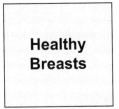

Ref: Eskin et al., Human Breast Uptake of Radioactive Iodine, *Obstetrics & Gynecology*, 1974.

Scientists have determined some specific actions of iodine on the breast.

- When dietary iodine was blocked in rodents, they developed swelling, nodules and benign breast disease.
- Rodents given the breast cancer-causing chemical, DMBA would not develop tumors if they were iodine-sufficient.
- Iodine desensitizes estrogen receptors in the breast.
- When scientists (Vega-Riveroll et al) gave a group of breast cancer patients iodine after

> biopsy, iodine (1) caused cancer cell death,
> (2) slowed cancer cell division and (3) reduced
> the size and number of tumor-promoting
> blood vessels, Iodine reduced estrogen
> production from overactive ovaries.

Can we reverse the Perfect Storm? Can we reduce the risk for breast cancer by reverse-engineering the three confluent forces that create this life-threatening disease?

The Iodine Solution means "take action." Arrest the perfect storm in its tracks. Nip iodine deficiency in the bud. Learn more. Don't wait.

More Iodine Stories

Meet SuAnn: Mole came off breast, breast inflammation no longer measurable, no breast cancer recurrence.

I have three success stories from using iodine:

I had a small mole/growth on my skin on top of my left breast implant. I painted it with Lugol's 2% occasionally over a two year period. It came off and now I don't have to worry about a mole becoming cancerous.

In 2009, I had a thermogram showing a hot spot on my right breast. Now annual thermograms do not show any inflammation on my right breast. I have been taking Iodoral with companion nutrients as well as painting my breast with Lugol's Iodine.

I also have NO recurrence of breast cancer on my left side since my mastectomy three years ago (Iodoral and Lugol's).

Meet Jo: Libido and ambition return.

The first day after taking 40 mg of Lugol's, I went to sleep experiencing a "weird" heartbeat and was thinking I would go back to 20 the next day because of that. But then I woke up having a sexy dream and was still "interested" when I woke up, which is really a big deal because I've had zero sex drive for some time now. Then I was able to make breakfast, take a shower, put on clothes, cross a busy street to mail a letter, and walk a mile to the pet store and back. Doesn't sound like much, but this is really a marked improvement. I'd been putting off doing these things for days, and today was the first day I had the ability.

Meet Felicia: Menopausal night sweats disappear.

My doctor told me iodine normalizes all the hormone receptors. Maybe this is why my menopausal night sweats have completely disappeared.

Meet Greg: Bleeding gums and gum pain resolve with Lugol's iodine flossing.

I believe I got rid of my bleeding and irritated (inflamed) gums by flossing with dental floss saturated in iodine. I've had this problem in varying degrees for over a year. With the saturated flossing thread, I got the iodine to the "root" of the problem. After just a couple of weeks with twice daily flossing all my pain and bleeding are gone. Now I'm off "iodine floss" and on normal floss in order to see if it returns or not. (Fingers crossed).

Meet Maddy: Post breast cancer cyst detected on mammogram vanishes.

I'm a 60 year-old cancer coach and a breast cancer survivor. I had breast cancer fifteen years ago and had a mastectomy on my left breast. Then, in 2008, I developed a cyst in my remaining breast.

It showed up big on a mammogram plus I could feel it. I was concerned it could turn into a recurrence so I tried several things. Nothing worked. On Lynne's Breast Cancer Think Tank I heard about Funahashi's work using iodine and progesterone in animals. His results showed progesterone helps drive iodine to the right cells. So I took 50 mg Iodoral by mouth and applied Lugol's Iodine with a Q-Tip over the cyst area of my breast and a dab of natural progesterone cream once the Lugol's absorbed into my skin.

The cyst began to shrink within 48 hours. So I dropped down on the Iodoral to 25 mg. Bad idea. The cyst came right back. After sticking with the protocol, the cyst went away. My doctor was no longer able to find anything on imaging. He wrote on the report that the cyst had disappeared. I gave all this documentation to Lynne—she uses my scan pictures in her slides when she speaks.

Meet Jane: Thyroid nodules and cysts no longer visible.

I can tell you that as of my last thyroid ultrasound, my thyroid nodules and cysts are no longer visible.

I won't have an ultrasound to look at my shrinking uterine fibroids for a while. As soon as I get some concrete evidence, and see the look on my ob/gyn's face, I will contact you.

Meet Marjorie: This is her story about her nickel-sized breast lump, fibromyalgia and other important observations (printed with permission from her blog).
http://thisissogood.wordpress.com/2012/02/10

This is another one of those posts that I have wanted to write for many months. Hopefully you find it interesting and maybe helpful to you or someone you know. My purpose is two-fold: discuss my experience with fibrocystic breast disease and iodine supplementation and review *Iodine Why You Need It and Why You Can't Live Without It.*

In 2005 (age 28), I found a small mass in my left breast. At the time I was completely wrapped up in the conventional wisdom mindset. Low fat and so-called "heart healthy" whole grains were in my regular rotation, I was clocking serious chronic cardio at the gym, and Western medicine seemed to have all the answers. Panicking, I called my physician and went in for a breast exam. She agreed that the mass was abnormal and immediately sent me for a mammogram. I was a stressed mess leading up to that test and during the mammogram, I almost passed out. I think it was a combination of the pain (OMG) and anxiety.

Sure enough, they saw something on the films! I was instructed to see a surgeon to discuss my options. He informed me that I had fibrocystic breast disease and that the mass I found was a fibroadenoma. Not cancerous, but something that should be removed because if left alone, they can grow to the size of softballs (more panicking). So I agreed to have it removed on an outpatient basis. I was awake during surgery, and he showed me the lump as he removed it. It was barely the size of a small marble. Off it went to be tested and a few days later I got the all clear call. Whew!

So, why did this happen? What do I do about it? Will I continue to undergo surgery after surgery as these show up in the future? Answers were in this order: We don't know, nothing—just watch it with regular mammograms, and, yes, you cannot ignore breast masses. Fabulous. So, like a good girl, I continued to have regular breast exams and routine mammograms plus numerous ultrasounds. During this time, there were no suspicious masses or lumps. After the second mammogram, I started to refuse. My Western medicine doctor agreed to let me stop them until I turned 40 as long as I did regular breast exams. OK. Deal.

Meanwhile, I had developed chronic low back pain. In 2009, I started to seek alternative treatment for my pain, as conventional medicine had failed to relieve my symptoms ... I had fantastic success with a Holistic physician and asked him for a referral to a Holistic family practice doctor. I was now a full blown believer in Alternative/Holistic/Naturopathic medicine. In April, 2011, I transferred all of my records to her office and saw her for a physical to establish myself as a patient. We discussed my fibrocystic breast disease history. She did an exam and noted no abnormalities, but stated we would watch from year-to-year (still encouraging me to do regular breast exams). One month later, I found a nickel sized mass in my right breast. Oh no—here we go again ... I made an appointment to see my new doctor and during the one week leading up to the appointment, the mass had increased in size (now approximately quarter-sized). Recalling all that was said to me in the past, I blabbered on to her about not wanting surgery or a mammogram! She listened and then quickly calmed my fears. Absolutely no mammograms and a very good chance that I could avoid surgery.

Step one was testing with breast thermology. Totally non-invasive, painless, and no, nothing—just watch it with regular mammograms, and yes, you cannot ignore radiation free. The procedure is not covered by insurance (of course), but I was willing to shell out the $100 for peace of mind and some answers to my current condition.... As expected, my scan came back negative for cancer, but positive for another fibroadenoma.

Step two was to start supplementing with high doses of Iodine (50 mg Iodoral) and 100 mcg Selenium. I don't know why, but this really freaked me out. The US RDA for Iodine is 150 mcg. Was it safe to take so much? What are the side effects? Would there be long term consequences?

My doctor assured me that there was no need to worry. Although I trusted her, I was still unsure. I hurried home and started to research Iodoral supplementation and fibrocystic breast disease. I found next to nothing. What I did find online was quite discouraging. Women reporting that they had tried Iodoral without improvements in their symptoms. At the same time all of this was occurring, Alex had a friend at work that was being treated for breast cancer by Dr. David Brownstein's Center for Holistic Medicine in West Bloomfield, MI. She purchased his book, *Iodine: Why You Need It and Why You Can't Live Without It*, for me, and I dug into it as soon as I got my hands on it. I won't get into the science here, I won't do it justice. What I will say is that the breasts and the thyroid are two of the body's main storage sites for Iodine. In a deficient or depleted state, these tissues become primed for illness including fibrocystic breast disease and breast cancer. Dr. Brownstein's book contains an entire chapter devoted to this topic.

So I decided to give the supplementation a try. My instructions were to take 50 mg Iodoral and 100 mcg Selenium one time a day for six weeks, and then cut the Iodoral in half to 25 mg (continue to take the Selenium) for another six weeks. After that, my physician said I could again cut the Iodoral dose in half (12.5 mg) and continue to take the selenium. This would be my maintenance dose.

I did it. And guess what? IT WORKED!!! Within a couple of weeks the mass was smaller, less dense, and not as tender. Within a month it was half the size it was before supplementation. Within two months, it was GONE. Gone—without pain, without stress, without an invasive procedure.

So why did it work? From Dr. Brownstein's book *Iodine: Why You need It and Why You Can't Live Without It*:

Animal studies have shown conclusively that an iodine deficient state can alter the structure and function of the breasts. After my own research and study, I concur with several investigators that iodine deficiency is a causative factor in breast cancer and fibrocystic breast disease. I believe it is essential that women have their iodine levels tested, and if it is shown there is an iodine deficiency, iodine supplementation should be initiated.

The breasts are one of the body's main storage sites for iodine in the body. In an iodine-deficient state, the thyroid gland and the breasts will compete for what little iodine is available. Therefore, this will leave the thyroid gland and the breasts iodine depleted and can set the stage for illnesses such as goiter, hypothyroidism, autoimmune thyroid disease, breast illnesses including cancer, and cystic breast disease. In addition, other glandular tissues such as the ovaries which contain the second highest concentration of iodine in the body, will also be depleted in an iodine deficient state.

The breasts and thyroid aren't the only utilizers of iodine. It is needed by the prostate gland, the gastrointestinal tract, salivary glands, bones, and connective tissues. If you have any of these parts and you want to keep them healthy, you should probably make sure you have adequate iodine in your diet.

So that's my story and I felt it was important to share. My fibrocystic breast disease was present way before I started a Paleo/Primal/Ancestral lifestyle, but I think it's valuable to note that this eating style is generally low in iodine. Most of us opt for Celtic sea salt over iodized table salt when cooking after we make the switch. Cutting out packaged, processed foods also cuts out iodized salt intake. Our soil, especially in the Mid-Western states, is deficient in Iodine, meaning our produce and pastured animal products are not a good source. Fish is a decent source, and sea vegetables are fabulous sources, but these are not foods that are typically eaten everyday by our population.

I strongly encourage you to find a Holistic or Naturopathic physician that can assist you in testing and determining your need for Iodine supplementation. I wouldn't recommend undertaking this on your own, as your doctor will likely want to monitor your thyroid function while supplementing.

There is one other note that I wanted to make. I work in the medical field and am nose deep in conventional Western medicine every day. I truly believe that there are Western medicine practices and amazing medical advancements that have improved our lives greatly. However, our current medical field does have its shortcomings and my story is an example. We should not be treating the symptoms, we should be investigating and treating the cause. Otherwise, are we truly ever healed or are we just chasing our tails?

Chapter Nineteen

Moving Forward—
Beyond the *Iodine Crisis*

Every truth passes through three stages before it is recognized.
In the first, it is ridiculed. In the second, it is opposed.
In the third, it is regarded as self-evident.

—Arthur Schopenhauer

You have finished reading *The Iodine Crisis*. What is next? By now, you are clearly aware of the problem, and awareness is always the first step in moving forward.

- What will your iodine journey be?
- Can you challenge the epidemic iodine crisis?
- Can you find a personal solution to this public health disaster?
- Can you explore the medical mystery of *who stole iodine*?
- Can you apply that solution to yourself?
- After reading all the life-altering case studies, can you craft your own plan?
- Can you launch your own iodine journey?

Join others learning about the iodine crisis and get started. Share your problem and your solution. Share the story of the

Chinese village where for 500 years the children wouldn't grow, where the goats miscarried. Share the story of the mom of three who couldn't get out of bed; the young man who finally was able to help out his family; or the women who got rid of the pain in their breasts.

Everyone who is helped by iodine builds the body of existing, positive research with their own personal experience. By sharing, we will defeat the Iodine Crisis. Because, while iodine deficiency is epidemic worldwide, the pain and isolation affects us individually—*one at a time. Sharing information is the only way.* Our boon for this process is the power of the Internet, available for the first time to the most recent generations of our troubled world. If just one person can be rescued from the abyss of a chronic complaint, sharing the information in The Iodine Crisis will be worth the time taken to read it.

Remember the disconcerting fact: most doctors and scientists cannot speak out directly against the current "standard of care" RDA iodine recommendations. Where has that thinking—that standard of care—come from? Not from facts, and not from people who have experienced the life changing iodine facts. Most licensed practitioners must play along with the old, mainstream thinking because the personal price for reporting positive, effective discoveries that challenge that thinking is too high.

We need to support the practitioners who are discreetly whistle-blowing about iodine deficiency. Unfortunately, discovery of an effective solution to a health problem can damage a career or jeopardize a license. History is filled with examples of conservative—no, reactionary—thinking standing in the way of important discoveries made by thoughtful, farsighted individuals—solutions to age-old problems causing untold suffering.

Remember, in the 1800s, Dr. Semmelweis was ridiculed for suggesting that doctors should wash their hands before delivering babies in order to prevent the mothers from dying of childbed fever.

What a paradox—the more a medical or scientific professional knows about life-changing information, the more he or she must hang back.

The privilege of spreading the word *falls* to the lay public of patient-to-patient medicine. The case studies we share here need to reach more people—need to be much more broadly publicized. As you have seen outlined in *The Iodine Crisis,* the steps for fixing the iodine crisis are available and have been for decades. I urge you to take the iodine information to your friends and family. Share the stories of scientists and practitioners who cannot because they are not in a position to popularize non-standard medical truths about iodine deficiency.

Writing as a journalist and a layperson makes it possible for me to say, "Look at the information my fellow travelers discovered." Fact-check them. Fact-check me. Learn. Test the information. No one can fire me for challenging the previous iodine groupthink. No one will shun me. *No one will shun you.* We know now, there are too many of us.

This book allowed me to share my passion for how iodine changed my life and the lives of many others. If you share my passion, please speak out. We must call for change. The stakes are too high to hang back.

- *Whistle blow!* The current recommended daily allowance for iodine is 150 mcg. That's too low for our current bromine-saturated environment. Contact The National Academy of Sciences and ask them to rethink their recommendations.
- *Reject it!* The much-promoted notion that iodized salt provides enough iodine for optimal health is a *complete scam!* Reject it. No one even knows how much iodine is actually in salt since it vaporizes out as soon as the carton is opened.

- *Share it!* Speak out about the pervasive presence of anti-iodine bromine-bromide additives in our foods and our environment, additives that may be a further underlying cause of the current Iodine Crisis.
- *Give it!* Give this book to your health practitioners. Tell them you want to start your own iodine experimentation.

I'm on the iodine information campaign for the long haul—in "for the duration." So are my friends in the Grass Roots Iodine Movement. We won't let the legacy of this movement slip away.

Visit *www.IodineResearch.com* for more information. Or visit me on *www.LynneFarrow.net*.

I will continue compiling iodine success stories to document the effects of individual usage.
If you have a personal story to report, please email me the details at *Lynne@LynneFarrow.net*

Part 4

Resources

Resource Listings

The Iodine Loading Test

Dr. Guy E. Abraham, with his colleagues, have found the 24 Hour Iodine Loading test helpful in assessing a patient's iodine sufficiency.

The principle is, if the body's level of iodine is adequate, most of the 50 mg iodine ingested at the start of the test will be excreted in the urine within 24 hours.

If the body shows insufficiency, a significant portion of the pre-test iodine dose will be retained by the body. The amount excreted in the urine will be low.

The Iodine Doctors find that any test result showing saturation lower than 90 percent suggests the patient is a candidate for iodine supplementation.

Update from the '07 Iodine Conference: Normal test results in the presence of known iodine-deficiency conditions such as thyroid disorders or breast disease may indicate an absorption defect with the Sodium Iodide Symporter (NIS) mechanism. In this case, the iodine given as part of the test may not get absorbed and pass through the body into the urine.

There may be a "false normal" test result. The doctors recommend supplementing with iodine for three months and then repeating the test. As the iodine supplementation improves the absorption, the test numbers should go lower (appropriate to the clinical condition), then steadily rise.

For Iodine Investigation Project participants, Breast Cancer Choices recommends testing at FFP Labs to assure consistency of results for our database. In New York, have your practitioner contact Doctors Data Lab. Be sure your test includes the 50 mg Iodoral or get the Iodoral tablets from your practitioner.

To order the Iodine-Loading Test, contact FFP labs at 877-900-5556 for the test kit. You may also email the lab at *ffp_lab@yahoo.com* to see if there is an Iodine Literate Practitioner in your area or whether Dr. Flechas can be assigned your test results.

http://cypress.he.net/~bigmacnc/drflechas/index.htm

Hakala Labs also does iodine testing and will ship the test to Europe. For a more detailed description of the Iodine Loading Test, please read *The Iodine/Iodide Loading Test* by Jorge Flechas, MD. It can be found *at www.vrp.com.*

Iodine Supplementation Protocol
(From the October 2007 Iodine Conference)

Physicians Guy Abraham, MD, David Brownstein, MD, and Jorge Flechas, MD, have treated more than 4,000 patients with iodine supplementation. The protocol below is suggested by their writings and lectures. We acknowledge with appreciation their pioneering research and generous contributions to the field of Iodine Therapy. See references below the protocol.

Iodine and Companion Nutrients

- 50 mg Iodoral minimum (may start with 12.5 mg).
- Some practitioners may recommend another form of iodine such as Lugol's solution. Iodoral is the Lugol's formula in tablet form especially designed to avoid gastric irritation.
- Vitamin C: 3,000 mg per day (more may be necessary to detox bromide).
- 300-600 mg magnesium oxide (Iodine Investigation Project participants prefer magnesium glycinate or magnesium citrate.)
- 200 mcg selenium. The selenomethionine version is preferred by many.
- 500 mg niacin (B3) twice a day (NOT niacinamide). Start lower to avoid flush. 100 mg Vitamin B2 three times a day. The ATP Cofactor may be used as an alternative.
- ½ teaspoon* unprocessed sea salt added to diet. (See reference on the following page.)
- ¼ teaspoon unprocessed salt in 8 oz. water twice a day as needed.
- A comprehensive vitamin and nutrition program.

- (February 2008) Dr. Guy Abraham cautions that "excess calcium supplementation (2,000-3,000 mg/day) has been the most common cause of poor response to iodine supplementation." *Vitamin Research News* Vol. 22. Number 2.
- Protocol Update 2009: Data gathered from the Breast Cancer Choices Iodine Investigation Project participants reports that The ATP CoFactors helps speed iodine absorption and normalize TSH levels.

Lugol's Iodine Solution Chart: Milligrams of Iodine per Drop

Lugol's content per drop	Iodine	Iodide	Total
2%	1.0 mg	1.50 mg	2.50 mg
3%	1.5 mg	2.25 mg	3.75 mg
5%	2.5 mg	3.75 mg	6.25 mg
7%	3.5 mg	5.25 mg	8.75 mg
10%	5.0 mg	7.50 mg	12.50 mg
15%	7.5 mg	11.25 mg	18.75 mg

*The additional ½ teaspoon of unprocessed salt added to the diet has been added by consensus of the main patient-to-patient groups and some of the Iodine Doctors after the Iodine Conferences. Be sure to read the Salt Loading Protocol and ask your doctor before implementing salt loading, additional salt or any medical strategy.

The Salt Loading Protocol

Iodine users often use the salt-loading protocol to clear bromide and many other detox symptoms. Salt has been used for over a hundred years by doctors to clear bromide symptoms.

Dr. William Shevin presented his Salt Loading Protocol at the February 2007 Iodine conference:

- ¼ teaspoon* unprocessed, unrefined salt dissolved in ½ cup warm water, then followed immediately with 12-16 oz pure water.
- Repeat in 30-45 minutes if needed. May repeat again until copious urination begins.
- Observe subjective response (usually within several hours).

Visit Dr. Shevin on the web at *www.DrShevin.com*. Be sure to read the Salt Loading Protocol and ask your doctor before implementing salt loading or any medical strategy.

Read Dr. David Brownstein's book, *Salt Your Way to Health*, 2nd edition available at *www.DrBrownstein.com*.

---

*Note our Iodine Investigation Project participants have found ½ teaspoon salt dissolved in water works faster than the ¼ teaspoon dosage.

Iodine Related Bromide and Toxin Detoxification Symptoms and Strategies

Iodine-related bromide symptoms may include but are not limited to:

eye lid twitching

foot twitching

tingling in hands or feet

dark thoughts (e.g., there is no reason to live)

depression (e.g., there is no reason to get out of bed)

anxiety

emotionality

mouth and tongue sores and cuts or "sore mouth"

"different" acne, "bromide acne," "acne-like eruptions" without "coniform." (Some iodine users found zinc helps bromide acne.)

skin "cuts"

hair loss

brain fog

leg and hip ache (feels like arthritis)

rash (bromaderma)

metallic taste

sinus ache

cherry angiomas

runny nose

headache

sedation

lethargy

odd swallowing sensation (reported in old medical literature as "swollen glottis")

body odor (bromos is Greek for stench)

unusual urine odor or color

dry mouth

urethral spasm, frequent urination (mistaken for
    urinary infection)
diarrhea
constipation
vision changes
irritability
increased salivation
dream changes
hormone changes
kidney pain
breast tenderness (transient symptom reported to resolve)

Many of the Breast Cancer Choices' Iodine Investigation Project registrants, Curezone Iodine Forum members and Yahoo Iodine Group members found the following suggestions helpful if iodine detox symptoms from bromide, dead bacteria and other toxins were uncomfortable. Consult your doctor before implementing the strategies below:

1. The Salt Loading Protocol has benefited many as the most effective way to flush toxins released by taking iodine.
2. Pulse-dosing Iodine. This means stopping iodine for 48 hours to rest the kidneys while continuing with the Companion Nutrients.
3. Taking vitamin C spread out throughout the day to bowel tolerance.
4. Taking the complete Iodine Companion Nutrients. Numerous testimonials prove The Iodine Companion Nutrients, including the ATP CoFactors, enhance cell detoxification.
6. Drinking more water. This cannot be emphasized enough.
7. According to iodine users with skin symptoms, adding 25 mg zinc often helps.

Appendix A

The Bromide Dominance Theory— How Competitive Inhibition Causes Iodine Deficiency

A bromide* dominance condition may develop when bromine, acquired through environmental, occupational, iatrogenic or dietary exposure, causes bromine levels in the body to rise high enough to inhibit iodine enzyme metabolism.

Iodine supplementation alters the competitive bromine-iodine relationship causing bromide excretion. Thus, bromide dominance is diminished and proper iodine enzyme metabolism may be restored.

In the toxic 21st Century, these questions must be raised:

- Would we have such a severe iodine deficiency without bromide dominance?
- If iodine deficiency is the underlying cause of many diseases, is bromide "the underlying cause of the underlying cause?"
- Is bromide dominance creating a public health crisis?

---

*Author's Note: Consider the terms iodine and iodide interchangeable unless the difference is relevant to the discussion such as the iodide in iodized salt. Similarly, the reader should consider the terms bromine and bromide interchangeable as we discuss the power of any bromine-related chemical to inhibit iodine.

Where Does Bromide Dominance Come From?

Bromide is an insidious additive used in many common products, and as a pesticide. Because of the sheer amount of bromine-related chemicals supplemented products, exposure to this man-made additive has caused a depletion of iodine in human populations. Studies in lab animals provide alarming evidence that even small amounts of bromide exposure can be toxic (1).

What products contain bromine/bromide?

Currently, bromide is found in pesticides (methylbromide), some bread products (potassium bromate), brominated vegetable oil that may be added to citrus-flavored drinks, hot tub cleansers, certain asthma inhalers and prescription drugs, plastic products, some personal care products and some fabric dyes.

Effects of Bromine on the Organs

Iodine depletion weakens the thyroid and other organs (2)(3)(4)(5)(6). In individuals where the bromide-iodine ratio is less, bromide may not be problematic.

Thyroid

Elevated bromide levels have been implicated in every thyroid disease, from simple hypothyroidism to auto-immune diseases to thyroid cancer. Malenchenko found *bromide levels 50 times higher in thyroid cancer than normal thyroid tissue* (7).

Rats fed even *the minimal amount of bromine expected to be encountered in the environment* underwent goiter-like changes (8), an arguable case of bromide dominance. In the FIRE project, exposing rats to the brominated flame retardant compound, bromocyclodecane, showed consistent effects on the thyroid hormone axis, including decreased T4. Thyroid gland cells have increased size and larger nuclei, indicating increased synthetic activity (9).

With enhanced intake of bromide, *fully one-third of the iodine content in the thyroids of rats was replaced by bromide* (10).

Skin

Skin biopsied from a woman who had been on bromide-containing sedatives for nearly four years found increased bromide in normal skin and three times that in an affected skin lesion (11).

An infant administered a syrup containing sodium bromide developed vegetative lesions on the face and scalp (12).

Technicians exposed to brominated compounds for prolonged periods developed multiple cherry angiomas on the trunk and extremities (13).

Mental

The psychiatry literature abounds with cases of elevated bromide levels being implicated in mental conditions from depression to schizophrenia (14)(15)(16). As Guy Abraham, MD, asks, "How many people with misdiagnosed bromism are currently treated with psychiatric drugs?" (17). Bromide was used to suppress women's sex drive in the 1950s.

Hearing

Potassium bromate, a bread additive, is known to cause renal damage and permanent deafness in animals and man (18). In the FIRE project, the most relevant effect on exposing rats to 28 days of the brominated flame retardant compound, tetrabromo-bisphenol-A, was hearing. Specifically, the lower frequency range was affected (19).

Kidneys

The ability of bromate to cause cancer, especially kidney cancer, is a significant health concern (20). The gene expression in kidneys in rats given a high dose—100-week potassium bromate—in their drinking water showed marked gene expression difference from the lower non-cancer dose. The high dose kidney gene expression resembled an adenoma-like expression pattern (21).

Bromines in Common Products

Bread

Potassium bromate as an additive to most commercial bread and baked goods probably provides the most egregious contribution to bromine overload in Western cultures.

Bromated flour is product "enriched" with potassium bromate. Some commercial bakers claim they use bromated flour because it yields dependable results, and it makes more elastic dough which can stand up to bread hooks and other commercial baking tools (22). However, Pepperidge Farm manages to use only un-bromated flour with excellent results.

Note on Banning Potassium Bromate in Bread

The UK banned bromate in bread in 1990. Canada banned bromate in bread in 1994 (23). Proposal P230 in Australia: Food Regulation Ministerial Council (FSANZ), still has not finalized its July 2007 proposal to mandate iodized salt in breads, breakfast cereals and biscuits.

Back in 1999, the Center for Science in the Public Interest petitioned the FDA to prohibit the use of potassium bromate, charging that the FDA has known for years that bromate causes cancer in lab animals, but has failed to ban it (24). As of September 2007, the US FDA responded to a Breast Cancer Choices inquiry with the statement, "Potassium bromate is still listed as a safe additive."

Water

When drinking water containing bromide is exposed to ozone, the bromate ion, a powerful oxidizing agent, is formed. Two recalls of drinking water involving bromate have occurred: Wegmann's "Food Your Feel Good About" spring water recall in 2006, and Coca-Cola's "Dasani" in 2004 (25).

Toothpaste, Mouthwash and Gargles

Potassium bromate is an antiseptic and astringent in toothpaste, mouthwash and gargles. Very toxic if taken internally. May cause bleeding and inflammation of gums in toothpaste (26).

Bromine in Flame Retardants

Flame retardants reduce the flammability of a wide variety of commercial and household products. Some brominated home retardants (BFRs) migrate from the products in which they are used and enter the environment and people via dust (27).

Personal Products and Some Cosmetics

Sodium bromate in products like permanent waves, hair dyes and textile dyes: Sodium bromate is in permanent wave neutralizers, hair dye material, and the textile dyeing process (28). Benzalkonium is used as a preservative in some cosmetics (29).

References

1. Vobecky, M., et al., "Interaction of Bromine with Iodine in the Rat Thyroid Gland at Enhanced Bromide Intake," *Biol Trace Elem Res*, 1996.

2. Velicky, J., et al., "The Effect of Bromide on the Ultrastructure of Rat Thyrocytes," *Ann Anat*, 2004.

3. Pavelka, S., et al., "Bromide Kinetics and Distribution in the Rat, II: Distribution of Bromide in the Body," *Biol Trace Res*, 2000.

4. Velicky, J., et al., "Long Term Action of Potassium Bromide on the Rat Thyroid Gland," *Acta Histochem*, 1998.

5. Velicky, J., et al., "Potassium Bromide and the Thyroid Gland of the Rat: Morphology and Immunochemistry," 1997.

6. Vobecky, M., et al., "Interaction of Bromine with Iodine in the Rat Thyroid Gland at Enhanced Bromide Intake," *Biol Trace Elem Res*, 1996.

7. Malenchenko, A. F., et al., "The Content and Distribution of Iodine, Chlorine and Bromide in the Normal and Pathologically Changed Thyroid Tissue," *Med Radiol*, 1984.

8. Velicky, J., et al., "Potassium Bromide and the Thyroid Gland of the Rat: Morphology and Immunochemistry, RIA and INAA Analysis," *Ann Anat*, 1997.

9. *www.credocluster.info*, Issue 6, July, 2006.

10. Vobecky, M., et al., "Interaction of Bromine with Iodine in the Rat Thyroid Gland at Enhanced Bromide Intake," *Biol Trace Elem Res*, 1996.

11. Hubner, K., et al., "Skin Bromide Content and Bromide Excretion in Bromoderma Tuberosum," *Arch Derm Res*, 1976.

12. Bel, S., et al., "Vegetant Bromoderma in an Infant," *Pediatric Dermatology*, 2001.

13. Cohen, A., et al., "Cherry Angiomas Associated with Exposure to Bromides," *Dermatology*, 2001.

14. Horowitz, B. Z., et al., "Bromism from Excessive Cola Consumption," *Clinical Toxicology*, 1997.

15. Levin, M., "Transitory Schizophrenia Produced by Bromide Intoxication," *Am J Psychiatry*, 1946.

16. *www.gulflink.osd.mil/library/randrep/pb_paper/mr1018.2chap10.html*

17. Abraham, G. E., "The Combined Measurement of the Four Stable Halides by the Ion-Selective Electrode Procedure Following Their Chromatographic Separation on a Strong Anion Exchange Resin: Clinical Application," *The Original Internist*, 2006.

18. Morizono, T., et al., "The Effects of Cetrimide and Potassium Bromate on the Potassium Ion Concentration in the Inner Ear Fluid of the Guinea Pig," *Physiol Bohemoslov*, 1988.

19. *www.credocluster.info*, Issue 6, 2006.

20. *www.rtctoc.com/bromate.htm*

21. Geter, D., et al., "Kidney Toxicogenomics of Chronic Potassium Bromate Exposure in F334 Male Rats," EIMS Meta Data Report, 2006.

22. *www.wisegeek.com*

23. *www.rtctox.com/bromate.htm*

24. *www.cspinet.org/new/bromide.htm*

25. *www.rtctox.com/bromate.htm*

26. *www.healthycommunications.com/hazards_of_cosmetics_by_carol_barzac95.html*

27. *www.credocluster.info*, Issue 6 2006.

28. *www.alibaba.com/catalog/11292709/sodium_bromate_99_5.html*

29. *www.gina.antczak.btinternet.co.uk/CU/CUHOME.htm*

Appendix B

Iodine and the Breast

What if there was one nutrient which ...?

1. Desensitized estrogen receptors in the breast.
2. Reduced estrogen production in overactive ovaries.
3. Reduced fibrocystic breast disease which often precedes breast cancer.
4. Caused cancer cell death, slowed down cell division, reduced blood vessel growth to tumors.
5. Caused more cell death than the chemo drug, Fluorouracil.
6. Prevented rats from getting cancer when they were fed the breast cancer causing toxin DMBA.

Research Suggests Some Breast Cancers May Be an Iodine Deficiency Disease

As iodine consumption has gone down, breast cancer rates have gone up. But the research goes far deeper, exploring the effects of iodine supplementation on breast disease and breast cancer. This important breakthrough has been in the research pipeline for years but only recently has found momentum. After sifting through 50 years of iodine research and corresponding with researchers around the world, the author reports that abnormal iodine metabolism, due either to *bromide dominance* in the environment or a dietary deficiency of iodine, must be addressed as part of a preventive and/or a therapeutic strategy.

Iodine deficiency is growing worse.

Iodine consumption by Americans has dropped 50 percent since the 1970s as breast cancer rates have risen (1). In the US Goiter Belt, where iodine in the soil is lower, breast cancer is higher (2).

By contrast, the incidence and severity of breast cancer are less in Japan than in Europe and the US, is attributable to the diet (3). Japanese women consume 25 times more dietary iodine than North American women and have lower breast cancer rates (4).

Meanwhile, since the 1970s, in the US and several other countries, iodine-blocking bromine chemicals have been added to flour, some sodas, and medications, exacerbating the iodine deficiency.

Fluoridated drinking water also depletes iodine absorption. Thus, as women consume less iodine and excrete more due to toxic elements, our risk for breast cancer grows (5).

Iodine and Benign Breast Disease

Blocking iodine in rats' food supply led to progressive, human-like fibrocystic disease (atypia, sclerosing, calcifications, dysplastic changes) as the rats aged (6). Iodine supplemention of patients with fibrocystic disease helped to resolve fibrosis and reduced breast size (7).

For women with painful breasts accompanying fibrocystic disease, iodine improved symptoms in more than 50 percent of the women who took 6.0 mg. of iodine for six months (8), and brown sea algae improved pain and nodularity in 94 percent of the women (9). From the authors' observations of the Iodine Investigation Project participants, depending on the kind of iodine agent used, painful breast symptoms have resolved in from 24 hours to three months.

Since benign breast disease increases the risk of breast cancer (10), and iodine improves fibrocystic disease, we at Breast Cancer Choices propose studies to see if iodine supplementation decreases the risk of getting breast cancer and the risk of recurrence.

Iodine and Breast Cancer

For breast patients, iodine's therapeutic mechanisms of action may be at least three-pronged: Hormonal (11), Biochemical (12-18), Genetic (19).

That is, iodine desensitizes the estrogen receptors, alters the chemical pathways as well as effects the genes, resulting in less cell growth, and causing an anti-tumor effect by causing apoptosis (programmed cell death) of malignant cells.

Iodine-rich seaweed exhibits an anti-cancer effect in rats and in the lab on human breast cancer cells.

Adding seaweed to rats' food delays the onset and number of rat mammary tumors (20, 21). And in the lab, mekabu seaweed causes plant-induced cell death in three kinds of human breast cancer cells. Mekabu had a stronger effect on the cells than the chemo drug, 5-fluorouracil (22).

Adding iodine to chemically-induced (DMBA) rat breast tumors, stops the growth of the tumors. Adding iodine plus medroxyprogesterone gave the highest level of response: the growth-suppressed tumors showed 100 percent times the iodine content than the full blown (nonsuppressed) tumors. The researchers suggest that the uptake of iodine was enhanced by medroxyprogesterone (23).

As David Brownstein, MD, phrased it, *"You cannot give breast cancer to rats that have sufficient iodine."*

In small, preliminary patient studies, using the screening iodine-loading test, breast cancer patients excreted less urinary iodine than healthy people, implying iodine-deficiency (24, 25).

The Breast Cancer Choices Iodine Investigation Project is currently following patients taking iodine to prevent recurrence. Most patients report no side effects. Some report a range of non-breast improvements such as change in thyroid status, ovarian cysts resolving, fibroids shrinking, improved energy, mood and mental clarity.

But be aware, some iodine takers report what we believe to be iodine detoxing bromide into the bloodstream causing symptoms of *bromism*.

According to a Department of Defense commissioned report, bromism symptoms can manifest as lethargy, depression, "dark" thoughts, "brain fog," constipation, leg and hip pain, acne, rashes and other symptoms. These side effects are usually reversible in 24 to 48 hours by discontinuing the iodine and allowing a short period of washout before restarting at a lower dose. Again, as stated above, unprocessed salt in water has relieved detox symptoms quickly by speeding up bromide detox through the kidneys. See Part 4. *Resources*, The Salt Loading Protocol.

References

1. "NHANES: National Health and Nutrition Survey showed iodine levels have declined 50% in the US. CDC National Center for Health Statistics." *CDC. gov 2000.*

2. Eskin, B. A., "Iodine and Mammary Cancer," *Advances in Experimental Medicine and Biology,* 1977; 91: 1977; 91: 293–304.

3. Kurihara, M., "Cancer Statistics in the World," Nagoya Univ. Press, Nagoya, pp. 80-81, 1984.

4. Aceves, C., et al., "Is Iodine a Gatekeeper of the Integrity of the Mammary Gland?," *Journal of Mammary Gland Biology and Neoplasia,* 2005.

5. Brownstein, D., *Iodine. Why You Need It. Why You Can't Live Without It,* 2nd Edition, Medical Alternative Press, 2006.

6. Krouse, T. B., et al., *Age-Related Changes Resembling Fibrocystic Disease in Iodine-Blocked Rat Breasts, Arch* Pathol Lab Med, 1979.

7. Ghent, W. R., et al., "Iodine Replacement in Fibrocystic Disease of the Breast," *Can J Surg,* 1993.

8. Kessler, J., "The Effect of Supraphysiologic Levels of Iodine in Patients with Cyclic Mastalgia," *The Breast Journal,* 2004.

9. Bezpalov, V. G., et al., "Investigation of the Drug 'Mamoclam' for the Treatment of Patients with Fibroadenomatosis of the Breast," *Vopr Onkol*, 2005.

10. Hartmann, L. C., et al., "Benign Breast Disease and the Risk of Breast Cancer," *N Engl J Med*, 2005.

11. Shah, N. M., et al., "Iodoprotein Formation by Rat Mammary Glands During Pregnancy and Early Postpartum Period," *Proc Soc Exp*, 1986.

12. Venturi, S., "Is There a Role for Iodine in Breast Disease?," *The Breast*, 2001.

13. Cann, S. A., et al., "Hypothesis: Iodine, Selenium, and the Development of Breast Cancer," *Cancer Causes Control*, 2000.

14. Smyth, P. P., "Role of Iodine in Antioxidant Defense in Thyroid and Breast Disease," *Biofactors*, 2003.

15. Coochi, M. et al., "A New Hypothesis of Bio-Chemical Cooperation?," *Prog Nutr*, 2000.

16. Thrall, K. D., "Differences in the Distribution of Iodine and Iodide in the Sprague-Dawley Rats," *J Toxicol Environ Health*, 1992.

17. Eskin, B. A., et al., "Different Tissue Responses for Iodine and Iodide in Rat Thyroid and Mammary Glands," *Biol Trace Elem Res*, 1995.

18. Ghent, W. R., et al., "Iodine Replacement in Fibrocystic Disease of the Breast," *Can J Surg*, 1993.

19. Eskin, B. A., et al., "Microarray Characterization of Iodine Metabolic Pathways in Breast Cancer," p. 379, 2006.

20. Teas, J. et al., "Dietary Seaweed (Laminaria) and Mammary Carcinogens in Rats," *Cancer Res*, 1984.

21. Funahashi, H., et al., "Wakame Seaweed Suppresses the Proliferation of 7,12-Dimethybenz(a)-Anthracene-Induced Mammary Tumors in Rats," *Jpn J Cancer Res*, 1999.

22. Funahashi, H., et al., "Seaweed Preventing Breast Cancer?," *Jpn J Cancer Res*, 2001.

23. Funahashi, H., et al., "Suppressive Effect of Iodine on DMBA-Induced Breast Tumor Growth in the Rat," *J Surg Oncol*, 1996.

24. Eskin, B. A., et al., "Identification of Breast Cancer by Differences in Urinary Iodine, Abstract Number 2150, Presentation AACR Conference," 2005.

25. Brownstein, D., *Iodine. Why You Need It. Why You Can't Live Without It*, 2nd Edition, Medical Alternative Press, 2006.

26. Cann, S. A., et al., "Hypothesis: Iodine, Selenium, and the Development of Breast Cancer," *Cancer Causes Control*, 2000.

27. Abraham, G. E., et al., "Evidence that the Administration of Vitamin C Improves a Defective Cellular Transport Mechanism for Iodine: A Case Report," *The Original Internist*, 2005.

28. Abraham, G. E., "The Safe and Effective Implementation of Orthoiodo-supplementation in Medical Practice," *The Orginal Internist*, 2004.

29. Brownstein, D., *Iodine. Why You Need It. Why You Can't Live Without It,* Fourth Edition, Medical Alternative Press, 2006.

30. Vega-Riveroll, L., Mondragón P., Rojas-Aguirre J., et al., "The antineoplasic effect of molecular iodine on human mammary cancer involves the activation of apoptotic pathways and the inhibition of angiogenesis," 2008.

Appendix C

Bromine/Bromide-Containing Products which Compete with Iodine

Bromated flour is one of the largest food exposures of bromine chemicals. Most breads contain potassium bromate used as a dough conditioner. Bromate is usually not labeled on baked products. Pepperidge Farm claims their bread contains no bromated flour.

Bromine Fire Retardants (BFRs) are being phased out but are available in many stores in carpets, mattresses, children's pajamas, some stuffed animals, car interiors, electronics, upholstered furniture, drapery and phones. BFRs are usually unlabeled.

Brominated Vegetable Oil (BVO) is found in some sodas, energy drinks, and other foods. Check labels.

If you are taking a prescription drug, you can go to *www.RXList.com* and type in, for example, the name, Atrovent, the asthma inhaler. Then look for the drug description. Notice the ingredient "Ipratropium bromide" which is in the trade name drug and the generics. The antidepressant, Celexa, contains Citalopram Hydrobromide which according to a pamphlet from the 1950s, was marketed as an anti-nymphomania drug.

Sources for more information on bromine-containing products:

www.CosmeticAnalysis.com,
www.EWG.org and *www.GoodGuide.com*

Bromine is a widely used hot tub cleaner.

Benzalkonium is widely used as a preservative in some cosmetics.

Hexadecyltrimethylammonium Bromide is used in some toilet bowl cleaners.

Also look for:

Acetyl Bromide
Ethylene di bromide
Benzyl Bromide
Allyl Bromide
N-Bromosuccinimide
5 Bromophthalide5
Cyanophthalide
2 Bromoethane
Sulfonic Acid Sodium Salt
Ethyl Bromide
N-Butyl Bromide
N-Propyl Bromide

Hexadecyltrimethylammonium Bromide is found in some brands of the following:

Facial Powder
Fabric Softener Sheets
Blush
Leave-In Conditioner
Shampoo
Bronzer
Eye Shadow
Shampoo Plus Conditioner
Hair Relaxer
Styling Mousse/Foam

Hair Care (General)
Facial Moisturizer/Treatment
Insect Bites/Stings
Facial Cleanser
Makeup (General)
Body and Foot Scrub
Acne Creams and Gels
Styling Gel/Lotion
All Purpose Cleaner
Toilet Bowl Cleaner

Centramonium bromide is widely found in some cosmetics, shampoos, hair conditioners, antiseptics and personal care compounds also known under the following names or abbreviations:

- cetab; cetyl trimethyl ammonium bromide;
- cetyltrimethylammonium bromide powder;
- 1-hexadecanaminium, n,n,n-trimethyl bromide;
- hexadecyltrimethylamine bromide;
- rimethylammonium bromide;
- n,n,n-trimethyl-1-hexadecanaminium bromide;
- bromide 1-hexadecanaminium, n,n,n-trimethyl;
- n,n,n-trimethyl- bromide 1-hexadecanaminium;
- 1hexadecanaminium, n,n,ntrimethyl, bromide;
- (1-hexadecyl) trimethylammonium bromide.

Myrtrimonium Bromide, AKA Tetradonium bromide is found in some cosmetics, Clearisil, and some toilet tissue.

Laurtrimonium Bromide, AKA Domiphen Bromide in found in some mouthwash or dental products.

Sodium Bromide is found in some permanent waves, hair dyes, fabric dyes.

Cetyltrimethylammonium Bromide is found in some nail and other personal products.

Lauryl Isoquinolinium Bromide is found in some deodorants.

Other names of bromine-based chemicals:

Isopropyl Bromide
Bromo Benzene
1,3-Dibromo – 5,5-dimethylhydantoin
Propionyl Bromide
Bromo Acetyl Bromide
Iso Butyl Bromide
M-Bromo Nitro Benzene
M - Bromo Aniline
Bromo anisole
Para Bromo Phenol
Pyridine Hydrobromide
Phosphorus Oxybromide
1,3 Dibromo Propane
4 Bromo Toluene
1,4 Dibromo butane
Phosphorus Tribromide
Tetra Bromo Phthalic Anhydride
Ortho bromo benzoic acid
1 Bromo Pentane
Methyl Bromide (With / Without Chloropicrin)
Ortho Bomo Benzonitrile
Para Bromo Benzo Nitrile
2 Bromopropionic Acid
1 Bromo 3 Chloro Propane
Potassium Bromide
Ammonium Bromide

Bromines in Common Products

Bread

Potassium bromate as an additive to most commercial bread and baked goods probably provides the most egregious contribution to bromine overload in Western cultures.

Bromated flour is product "enriched" with potassium bromate. Some commercial bakers claim they use bromated flour because it yields dependable results, and it makes more elastic dough which can stand up to bread hooks and other commercial baking tools (1). However, Pepperidge Farm manages to use only unbromated flour with excellent results.

Note on Banning Potassium Bromate in Bread

The UK banned bromate in bread in 1990. Canada banned bromate in bread in 1994 (2). Proposal P230 in Australia: Food Regulation Ministerial Council (FSANZ), still has not finalized its July 2007 proposal to mandate iodized salt in breads, breakfast cereals and biscuits.

Back in 1999, the Center for Science in the Public Interest petitioned the FDA to prohibit the use of potassium bromate, charging that the FDA has known for years that bromate causes cancer in lab animals, but has failed to ban it (3).

As of September 2007, the US FDA responded to Breast Cancer Choices inquiry with the statement, "Potassium Bromate is still listed as a safe additive."

Water

When drinking water containing bromide is exposed to ozone, the bromate ion, a powerful oxidizing agent, is formed. Two significant recalls of drinking water involving bromate have occurred: Wegmann's "Food You Feel Good About" spring water recall in 2006, and Coca-Cola's "Dasani" in 2004 (4).

Toothpaste, Mouthwash and Gargles

Potassium bromate is an antiseptic and astringent in toothpaste, mouth and gargles. Very toxic if taken internally. May cause bleeding and inflammation of gums in toothpaste (5).

Bromine in Flame Retardants

Flame retardants reduce the flammability of a wide variety of commercial and household products. Some brominated home retardants (BFRs) migrate from the products in which they are used and enter the environment and people via dust (6).

Personal Products and Some Cosmetics

Sodium bromate in Products: Permanent Waves, Hair Dyes, Textile Dyes. Sodium bromate is in permanent wave neutralizers, hair dye material, and the textile dyeing process (7). Benzalkonium is used as a preservative in some cosmetics (8).

Breast Cancer Choices is indebted to the pioneering bromide research of Guy E. Abraham, MD, as well as the clinical and intellectual contributions of David Brownstein, MD, and Jorge Flechas, MD.

Consider the terms iodine and iodide interchangeable unless the difference is relevant to the discussion such as the iodide in iodized salt.

Similarly, the reader should consider the terms bromine and bromide interchangeable as we discuss the power of any bromine-related chemical to inhibit iodine.

References

1. *www.wisegeek.com*
2. *www.rtctox.com/bromate.htm*
3. *www.cspinet.org/new/bromide.htm*
4. *www.rtctox.com/bromate.htm*
5. *www.healthy-communications.com/hazards_of_cosmetics_by_carol_barzac 95.html*
6. *www.credocluster.info*, Issue 6 2006.
7. *www.alibaba.com/catalog/11292709/sodium_bromate_99_5.html*
8. *www.gina.antczak.btinternet.co.uk/CU/CUHOME.htm*

Appendix D

Fluoride in Pharmaceuticals which Compete with Iodine

Appendix D is by Heidi Stevenson, reprinted by permission. Visit her blog at: *Gaia-Health.com/gaia-blog/*

Author's note: do not discontinue any pharmaceutical without consulting your doctor.

Fluorine is a poison with no place in any living metabolism. Yet, it's commonplace in pharmaceuticals. See this list below of drugs containing fluorine.

Fluorine is a poison. It has no place in the metabolism of humans, animals, or plants. It destroys bones and teeth, and wreaks havoc on all body systems. Fluorine is one of the most pervasive elements in pharmaceutical drugs.

Modern, drug-based medicine depends on fluorine. Early symptoms of poisoning are generally not recognized, as they are commonly experienced. These can include excess salivation, nausea, vomiting, diarrhea, and abdominal pain. One must wonder how many people believe they have flu when they're actually suffering from fluorine poisoning.

These symptoms are insidious because they can indicate the beginnings of severe metabolic disorders that lead to endocrinological diseases, such as hypocalcemia, hypomagnesemia, hyperkalemia, and hypoglycemia. These conditions can have knock-on effects throughout the body in chronic disorders. Subclinical imbalances in any of these necessary substances—calcium, magnesium, potassium, and sugar—can result in long term and permanent harm.

Fluorine poisoning can also result in neurological damage, including headaches, tremors, spasms, tetanic contractions, hyperactive reflexes, seizures, and muscle weakness. Ultimately, it causes teratogenic disorders—birth defects of the worst sort.

It is, in fact, fluorine that makes dioxins so horrific. (For information about dioxin poisoning in the United States, along with a photo gallery of deformities that its incarnation as Agent Orange in Vietnam unleashed, and its effects on children in England, search the web.

Cardiovascular involvement can result in widening of QRS (abnormality in heartbeat that can result in sudden death), arrhythmias, shock, and cardiac arrest.

Many common, and many infamous, drugs contain fluorine:

Prozac, the first SSRI.
Flonase, decongestant.
Lipitor and Baycol, cholesterol reducers.
Diflucan, antifungal drug.
Cipro, antibiotic.
Prevacid and Propulsid, antacids.

This list goes on … and on and on.

Ingesting a drug with fluorine is a risky act. You might think that special warnings would be placed on drugs compounded with fluorine, but none are.

To help you protect yourself, here's a list of most of the fluorine-based drugs, broken down by their typical use. The list is by generic name. If the drug has been removed from the market, the year is added in parentheses.

Drugs Which Contain Fluorine

Anesthetics
Desflurane
Droperidol
Enflurane
Flumazenil
Halophane
Isoflurane
Methoxyflurane
Midazolam
Sevoflurane

Antacids
Lansoprazole
Cisapride (2000)

Anti-anxiety
Flurazapam
Halazepam
Hydroflumethiazide

Antibiotics (Fluoroquinolones)
Ciprofloxacin
Penetrex
Flucloxacillin
Gatifloxacin
Gemifloxacin mesylate
Grepafloxacin HCI
Levofloxacin
Linezolid
Lomefloxacin
Moxifloxacin HCl
Norfloxacin
Sparfloxacin
Temafloxacin (1992)
Trovafloxacin mesylate

Antidepressants
Citalopram
Escitalopram
Prozac
Luvox
Paroxetine
Progabide

Antifungals
Fluconazole
Flucytosine/Voriconazole

Antihistamines
Astemizole
Levocabastine (1999)

Antilipemics (Cholesterol Lowering)
Atorvastatin
Cerivastatin sodium (2003)
Ezetimibe
Fluvastatin sodium

Antimalarial
Halofantrine
Mefloquine

Antimetabolites (Chemotherapy)
Aprepitant
Fluorouracil

Antipsychotics
Fluphenazine HCI
Haloperidol
Trifluoperazine HCI

Rheumatoid Arthritis
Celecoxib
Diflunisal
Flurbiprofen
Leflunomide
Sulindac

Steroids
Amcinonide
Betamethosone diproprionate
Clobetasol
Clocortolone
Dexamethasone
Diflorasone
Dutasteride
Flumethasone Pivalate
Flunisolide
Fluocinolone Acetonide
Fluocinonide
Fluorometholone
Fluticasone propionate
Flurandrenolide
Hydroflumethiazide

Iodine Glossary

Atomidine — A liquid iodine preparation also called detoxified iodine. Reputed to have been invented by Edgar Cayce.

ATP Cofactors — A specific dosage, vitamin product developed by Optimox to enhance iodine absorption.

Breast Cancer Choices' Iodine Investigation Project — The database created to assess the urinary iodine values in breast cancer patients who take the Iodine Loading Test.

Bromaderma — Skin rash sometimes caused by exposure to or consumption of bromine or bromide products.

Bromated flour — The main flour used in the Western world since the 1970s when potassium iodate, a crucial source of dietary iodine, was removed from flour. Bromated flour contains potassium bromate as a dough conditioner.

Bromine — The chemical element in the halogen family which competes with iodine for the halogen receptors in the body. Bromine chemical compounds are most often found as potassium bromate in wheat flour or Brominated Vegetable Oil (BVO) in foods and soft drinks. PBDE fire retardants contain the bromine compound **polybrominated diphenyl ethers** or **PBDEs**. PBDEs have been used in a wide array of products, including building materials, electronics, furnishings, motor vehicles, airplanes, plastics, foams, and textiles. They are structurally akin to the better known PCBs.

Bromide detox — The detoxification flow of bromine products from the body tissues to the bloodstream when exposed to salt or displaced by iodine into the urine as bromide.

Bromide Dominance Theory — The hypothesis conceived from the investigation and scholarship developed by Lynne Farrow positing iodine deficiency may be, in part, a man-made condition created by the addition of bromine products into foods and fire retardants since the 1970s:

> *A bromide dominance condition may develop when bromine, acquired through environmental, occupational, iatrogenic or dietary exposure, causes bromine levels in the body to rise to a high enough level to inhibit iodine enzyme metabolism. Iodine supplementation alters the competitive bromine-iodine relationship causing bromide excretion. Thus, bromide dominance is diminished and proper iodine enzyme metabolism may be restored.*

Bromism — The toxic state of excessive amounts of bromine building up in the tissues or bloodstream.

Curezone Iodine Forum — One of the original online iodine user groups exchanging of up-to-date research on both the using, history and science of iodine. The forum has many long-time contributors from all over the world and has produced a rich database of trial and error iodine experiences. As of January 2013, the forum had received over 15 million page views.

Dr. Abraham Effect — The urge to accumulate iodine research and history after reading the works of Guy E. Abraham, MD. This urgency is a newly discovered auto-regulatory mechanism found in the frontal lobe of the brain occurring after iodophobia-remission has been achieved.

Fibrocystic breast disease — An umbrella term describing swelling, cysts, nodules, scar tissue, fibrous tissue or breast pain.

Funahashi Method — The name given to a patient-initiated technique for reducing breast cysts. The method involves applying Lugol's Iodine to the breast topically along with five mg progesterone cream in addition to 50 mg Lugol's Iodine or Iodoral. This technique has nothing to do with Dr. Funahashi, who achieved good results in rodents combining progesterone and iodine. As with any other medical procedure, check with your licensed health care professional.

Goitrogen — Any substance, microbe or food that suppresses thyroid function.

Grass Roots Iodine Movement — The patient to patient education movement arising after Drs. Abraham, Brownstein and Flechas published their findings about the benefits of iodine. Once the information was leaked to influence leader groups, patient-to-patient research and experimentation commenced that ignited a mass sharing of information. The dramatic beneficial results of iodine supplementation created a word of mouth revolution that challenged the previous belief in the Wolff-Chaikoff Effect.

Iodide — A form of the chemical element, iodine, widely used as potassium iodide in iodized salt as well as medicines, and as a protection from radiation exposure.

Iodine — An element in the halogen family discovered by Bernard Courtois in 1811. Iodine is essential to human and animal function. Thus, iodine and its compounds are used in nutrition. Seaweed was one of the first known sources of iodine for human health. In the mid 1800s iodine became widely regarded as a "universal medicine."

Iodine "Boing" — The nickname for the jolt of mental clarity some iodine takers report when beginning iodine supplementation.

Iodine Companion Nutrients — See Iodine Protocol in Part 4. *Resources.*

Iodine Denier — **1.** A person who denies that tens of thousands of people have radically improved their health by supplementing iodine via the guidelines established by the Iodine Project. **2.** A person who claims iodine supplementers are at grave risk if they persist in this folly. **3.** A person who attempts to discredit iodine supplementation because he does not support the religious beliefs of the primary investigator. **4.** A person who maintains belief in the Wolff-Chaikoff Effect after it has been disputed.

Iodine Workshop on Facebook — The online group founded by *IodineResearch.com* editor Lynn Razaitis and frequented by the author.

Iodine Literate Practitioner — See Iodine Literate Practitioner Directory for full description.

Iodine Loading Test — The 24 hour urine collection test developed to assess iodine sufficiency.

Iodine Project — The iodine research group which began publishing their findings in 2002 under the leadership of Guy E. Abraham, MD.
    See *http://www.optimox.com/pics/Iodine/IOD-08/IOD_08.htm*

Iodine Resistance — A general term coined to investigate and identify what factors may inhibit iodine absorption.

Iodoral — The Lugol's iodine tablet manufactured by Optimox.

Lugol's Iodine Solution — The iodine product developed by Dr. Jean Lugol in France in 1829. The solution consists of potassium iodide (KI) and elemental iodine (I2). The potency of the solution may vary depending on the concentration. The customary solution is 5%, but 2% and 7% are available.

NAI Symporter — Stands for sodium iodide symporter. The symporters are tissues used by the body to trap iodine from the bloodstream. Unfortunately, over time the "traps" can become damaged by pollutants and oxidation (think rust) or become scarce. Atrophied symporters can worsen an iodine deficiency. In order to heal, iodine is necessary in combination with antioxidants.

Oxidative Damage — Damage to tissues such as iodine symporters from anti-oxidant starvation.

Post scarcity effect — A theory explaining the body's adaptation to a sudden increased iodine supply after a period of iodine scarcity. Can be manifested as breasts or thyroid swelling to trap and hoard more iodine from the bloodstream in anticipation of another period of scarcity. Think squirrels collecting acorns for the winter.

Potassium Bromate — An additive to bread and other baked goods which replaced iodine in the 1970s. The replacement of potassium iodate with potassium bromate is thought to be in part responsible for the World Health Organization's finding that we excrete 50 percent less iodine than we did 30 years ago.

Pulse dosing — The 48-hour interrupted iodine dosing strategy developed by Breast Cancer Choices' Iodine Investigation project. The regimen includes stopping daily iodine usage temporarily, usually for 48 hours, to enhance detoxification by rest; the rest strengthens the organs' ability to clear any bromides, microbes or toxins. Pulse dosing is generally used only when detoxification becomes uncomfortable. The salt loading protocol is suggested during the 48 hour iodine "fast."

Salt Loading Protocol — Part of the iodine protocol that entails taking specific amounts of salt and water to facilitate the detoxification process. This procedure is a variation of an old remedy used in medicine as well as by the US Army after the certain soldiers were diagnosed with bromide toxicity.

SSKI — Saturated solution of potassium iodide.

Stealth Bromide — Bromide exposure that is not labeled, such as the bromine fire retardants (BFRs) in our mattresses, furniture, carpeting, electronics, upholstery, toys, cars and children's pajamas. Many personal care products from cosmetics to permanents also contain chemicals in the bromine family.

The Perfect Storm Theory of Breast Cancer — The hypothesis created by the author, Lynne Farrow, suggesting the increases incidence of certain cancers, specifically, breast and thyroid cancers, since 1970, may be a result of a confluence of events in which iodine consumption dropped by 50 percent and bromide exposure began to saturate the environment with bromine fire retardants and other bromide toxins.

Wolff-Chaikoff Effect — The influential theory which gained dominance in the last 50 years positing that iodine shuts down the thyroid in rats. Wolff-Chaikoff has since been challenged.

Additional References and Resources

Abernathy, et al., "Polybrominated diphenyl ethers in maternal and fetal blood samples." *Environmental Health Perspectives*, July 1, 2003.

Abraham G. E., "The Combined Measurement of the Four Stable Halides by the Ion-Selective Electrode Procedure Following Their Chromatographic Separation on a Strong Anion Exchanger Resin: Clinical Applications." *The Original Internist*, 171-195, December, 2006.

Abraham, G. E., et al., "Evidence that the Administration of Vitamin C Improves a Defective Cellular Transport Mechanism for Iodine: A Case Report." *The Original Internist,* 2005.

Abraham, G. E., Flechas, J. D., Hakala, J. C., "Optimum Levels of Iodine for Greatest Mental and Physical Health." *The Original Internist*, 9:5-20, 2002.

Abraham, G. E., Flechas, J. D., Hakala, J. C., "Orthoiodosupplementation: Iodine Sufficiency of the Whole Human Body." *The Original Internist*, 9:30-41, 2002.

Abraham, G. E., Flechas, J. D., Hakala, J. C., "Measurement Of Urinary Iodide Levels By Ion-Selective Electrode: Improved Sensitivity And Specificity By Chromatography On An Ion-Exchange Resin." *The Original Internist*, 11(4):19-32, 2004.

Abraham, G. E., "The Wolff-Chaikoff Effect: Crying Wolf?" *The Original Internist*, 12(3):112-118, 2005.

Abraham, G. E., "The safe and effective implementation of orthoiodosupplementation in medical practice." *The Original Internist*, 11:17-36, 2004.

Abraham, G. E., "The concept of orthoiodosupplementation and its clinical implications." *The Original Internist*, 11(2):29-38, 2004.

Abraham, G. E., "Serum inorganic iodide levels following ingestion of a tablet form of Lugol solution: Evidence for an enterohepatic circulation of iodine." *The Original Internist*, 11(3):112-118, 2005.

Abraham, G. E., "The historical background of the iodine project." *The Original Internist*, 12(2):57-66, 2005.

Abraham, G. E., Brownstein, D., "Evidence that the administration of Vitamin C improves a defective cellular transport mechanism for iodine: A case report." *The Original Internist*, 12(3):125-130, 2005.

Abraham, G. E., "Brownstein, D., Flechas, J. D., The saliva/serum iodide ratio as an index of sodium/iodide symporter efficiency." *The Original Internist*, 12(4):152-156, 2005.

Abraham, G. E, MD, "The History of Iodine in Medicine Part I: From Discovery to Essentiality." *The Original Internist*, 13:29-36, Spring, 2006.

Abraham, G. E., "The History of Iodine in Medicine Part II: The Search for and the Discovery of Thyroid Hormones." *The Original Internist*, 13:67-70, June, 2006.

Abraham, G. E., "The History of Iodine in Medicine Part III: Thyroid Fixation and Medical Iodophobia." *The Original Internist*, 13:71-78, June, 2006.

Abraham, G. E, MD, and Flechas, J. D., MD, "Evidence of Defective Cellular Oxidation and Organification of Iodide in a Female with Fibromyalgia and Chronic Fatigue." *The Original Internist*, Vol. 14, 77-82, 2007.

Abraham, G. E, MD, and Flechas, J. D., MD, "The Effect of Daily Ingestion of 100 mg Iodine Combined with High Doses of Vitamins B2 and B3 (ATP Cofactors) in Five Subjects with Fibromyalgia." *The Original Internist*, Vol. 15, No. 1, pp. 8-15, March, 2008.

Abraham, G. E., MD, "Facts about Iodine and Autoimmune Thyroiditis." *The Original Internist*, Vol. 15, No. 2, pp. 75-76, June, 2008.

Aceves, C., et al., "Is Iodine a Gatekeeper of the Integrity of the Mammary Gland?" *Journal of Mammary Gland Biology and Neoplasia*, 2005.

Barkley, R. A., and Thompson, T. G., "The Total Iodine and Iodine-iodate Content of Sea Water." *Deep Sea Research* Vol. 7, Pergamon Press, London, 1960.

Bel, S., et al., "Vegetant, Bromoderma in an Infant." *Pediatric Dermatology*, 2001.

Bezpalov, V. G., et al., "Investigation of the Drug 'Mamoclam' for the Treatment of Patients with Fibroadenomatosis of the Breast." *Vopr Onkol*, 2005.

Brown-Grant and Rogers, "The Sites of Iodide Concentration in the Oviduct and the Uterus of the Rat." *Journal of Endocrinology*," 1972.

Brownstein, D., *Iodine. Why You Need It. Why You Can't Live Without It*, Editions 1-4, Medical Alternative Press, Michigan, 2006.

Brownstein, D., *Overcoming Thyroid Disorders*, Medical Alternatives Press, 2008.

Brownstein, D., "Clinical experience with inorganic, non-radioactive iodine/iodide." *The Original Internist*, 12(3):105-108, 2005.

Brownstein, D., multiple DVDs, *www.drbrownstein.com*.

Brownstein, D., *Natural Way to Health* newsletter, various issues, *newsmax.com*.

Buist, Stephanie, "My Journey Through Thyroid Cancer," *http://ds-ladybugsand-bees.blogspot.com/*.

Buist, Stephanie, "My Thyroid Cancer Story," *http://www.naturalthyroidchoices.com/MyStory.html*.

Cann, S. A., et al., "Hypothesis: Iodine, Selenium, and the Development of Breast Cancer." *Cancer Causes Control*, 2000.

Chilean Iodine Educational Bureau, *Geochemistry of Iodine: Annotated Bibliography 1825-1954*, London, 1956.

Chilean Iodine Educational Bureau, *Geochemistry of Iodine: Iodine in Rocks, Minerals and Soils, Annotated Bibliography 1825-1954*, London, 1956.

Chilean Nitrate Producers Association, Iodine Department, *Iodine for Farm Animals*, (pamphlet) October 30th, 1930, London.

Cogswell, C., AB, MD, "An Experimental Essay on the relative Physiological and Medicinal Properties of Iodine and its Compounds," Harveian Prize Dissertation for 1837. Medical Review, Quarterly. *Journal, Practical Medicine and Surgery*, Vol. 5, Jan-April, 1838, London.

Cohen, A., et al., "Cherry Angiomas Associated with Exposure to Bromides." *Dermatology*, 2001.

Dach, J., "Iodine Treats Breast Cancer, Overwhelming Evidence." *http://jeffrey dach.com/2009/11/13/iodine-against-breast-cancer-the-overwhelming-evidence-by-jeffrey-dach-md.aspx?ref=rss*.

Dillehay, T. D., *The Settlement of the Americas*, Basic Books, New York, 2000.

Dillehay, et al., "Monte Verde: Seaweed, Food, Medicine, and the Peopling of South America." *Science*, 320 (5877), pp. 784-786. May 9, 2008.

Dillehay, et al., "Plant Use Schedules," "Decreased Mobility," and "Social Differentiation: Hunter-Gatherers in Forested Chile," *Hunters and Gatherers in Theory and Archaeology*, edited by George M. Crothers, pp. 316-339. Occasional Paper No. 31. Center for Archaeological Investigations, Southern Illinois University, Carbondale, 2004.

Dasgupta, P. K., et al., "Iodine Nutrition: Iodine Content of Iodized Salt in the United States," *Environmental Science & Technology*, Vol. 42, No. 4, 2008.

DeLong, R., Robbins, J., Condliffe, P. G., *Iodine and the Brain*, Plenum Press, New York, 1989.

Dobson, J., "The Iodine Factor in Health and Evolution." *Geographical Review*, Vol. 88, 1998.

Eskin, B. A., et al., "Identification of Breast Cancer by Differences in Urinary Iodine." Abstract Number 2150, Presentation AACR Conference, 2005.

Eskin, B. A., et al., "Microarray Characterization of Iodine Metabolic Pathways," *Breast Cancer*, 2006.

Eskin, B. A., "Iodine and Mammary Cancer." *Adv Exp Med Biol*, 1977; 91:293-304

Eskin, B. A., et al., "Different Tissue Responses for Iodine and Iodide in Rat Thyroid and Mammary Glands." *Biol Trace Elem Res*, 1995.

Eskin, B. A., et al., *Human Breast Uptake of Radioactive Uptake, Obstetrics and Gynecology*, Harper and Row, New York, 1974.

Eskin, B. A., "Iodine Conference presentations," 2007.

Fernandez, Renate Lellep, *A Simple Matter of Salt: An Ethnography of Nutritional Deficiency in Spain*, Berkeley: University of California Press, 1990.

Flechas, Jorge, "Orthoiodinesupplementation in a Primary Care Practice." *The Original Internist*, 12(2):89-96, 2005.

Flechas, Jorge, "Iodine Conference presentations," 2007.

Funahashi, H., et al., "Seaweed Preventing Breast Cancer?" *Jpn J Cancer Res*, 2001.

Funahashi, H., et al., "Suppressive Effect of Iodine on DMBA-Induced Breast Tumor Growth in the Rat." *J Surg Oncol*, 1996.

Funahashi, H., et al., "Wakame Seaweed Suppresses the Proliferation of 7,12-Dimethybenz(a)-Anthracene-Induced Mammary Tumors in Rats." *Jpn J Cancer Res*, 1999.

Gardner, R. W., and Gardner, E. W., *The Applications of Iodine*, 1907.

Geter, D., et al., "Kidney Toxicogenomics of Chronic Potassium Bromate Exposure in F334 Male Rats." *EIMS Meta Data Report*, 2006.

Ghent, W. R., et al., "Iodine Replacement in Fibrocystic Disease of the Breast." *Can J Surg*, 1993.

Golumb, B. A., *A Review of the Scientific Literature As It Pertains to Gulf War Illnesses, Volume 2: Pyridostigmine Bromide*, The Rand Corporation, 1999.

"Grizz," iodine activist's compilation of sources. *http://tinyurl.com/iodine-references*.

Gugliotta, G., "Washington Post Georgrapher suggests Neanderthals were just Cretins," 1999. *http://www.trussel.com/prehist/news125.htm*.

Hartmann, L. C., Sellers, T. A., Frost, M. H., et al., "Benign breast disease and the risk of breast cancer." *N Engl J Med*. 2005; 353:229-237.

Hartmann, L. C., et al., "Benign Breast Disease and the Risk of Breast Cancer." *N Engl J Med* 2005; Shah, N. M., et al., "Iodoprotein Formation by Rat Mammary Glands During Pregnancy and Early Postpartum Period." *Proc Soc Exp*, 1986.

Hayden, D., *Pox: Genius, Madness and the Mysteries of Syphilis*, Basic Books, 2003.

Horowitz, B. Z., et al., "Bromism from Excessive Cola Consumption." *Clinical Toxicology*, 1997.

Hubner, K., et al., "Skin Bromide Content and Bromide Excretion in Bromoderma Tuberosum." *Arch Derm Res*, 1976.

"Ion Concentration in the Inner Ear Fluid of the Guinea Pig." *Physiol Bohemoslov*, 1988.

Jarvis, N. D., *Iodine Content of Pacific Coast Seafoods*, University of Washington College of Fisheries, University of Washington Press, Vol. 1, No. 12, November, 1928.

Kapdi, C., C., and Wolfe, J. N., "Breast Cancer: Relationship to Thyroid Supplement for Hypothyroidism." *JAMA*, Sept 6, 1976-Vol. 236, No. 10.

Kelly, F. C., "Iodine in medicine and pharmacy since its discovery—1811-1961." *Proc R Soc Med* 54, 831-836, 1961.

Kessler, J., "The Effect of Supraphysiologic Levels of Iodine in Patients with Cyclic Mastalgia." *The Breast Journal*, 2004.

Krouse, T. B., et al., "Age-Related Changes Resembling Fibrocystic Disease in Iodine-Blocked Rat Breasts." *Arch Pathol Lab Med*, 1979.

Kurihara, M., "Cancer Statistics in the World," Nagoya Univ. Press, Nagoya, pp. 80-81 1984.

Levin, M., "Transitory Schizophrenia Produced by Bromide Intoxication," *Am J Psychiatry*, 1946.

Lichtensteiger, W., et al., "Developmental Exposure to PBDE 99 and PCB affects estrogen sensitivity of target genes in rat brain regions and female sexual behavior." *Organohalogen Compounds*, Volume 66, 2004.

Lunder, S., and Sharp, R., *Tainted Catch.* The Environmental Working Group, 2003.

Lugol, Jean Guillaume Auguste, *Essays on the Effects of Iodine in Scrofulous Diseases*, translated from the French by William Brooke O'Shaunessy, 1831.

Madsen, T., Lee, S., and Olle, T., "Growing Threats: Toxic Flame Retardants and Children's Health." Editorial, *San Francisco Chronicle*, June 11, 2003.

Malenchenko, A. F., et al., "The Content and Distribution of Iodine, Chlorine and Bromide in the Normal and Pathologically Changed Thyroid Tissue." *Med Radiol*, 1984.

Masten, S., "Gum Guggal and Some of its Steroidal Constituents, National Toxicology Program," NIESH. *NIH*, 2005.

Meerts, I. A. T. M., et al., "In Vito Estrogenicity of Polybrominated Diphenyl Ethers, Hydroxylated PBDEs, and Polybrominated Bisphenol A Compounds." *Environmental Health Perpectives*, Vol. 109, Number 4, April, 2001.

NHANES: National Health and Nutrition Survey showed iodine levels have declined 50% in the US. CDC National Center for Health Statistics. *CDC. Gov*, 2000.

Olsson, L., *http://iodinehistory.blogspot.com/*.

Pandav, C. S., and Rao, R., *Iodine Deficiency Disorders in Livestock: Ecology and Economics*, Oxford University Press, England, 1997.

Pandav, C.S., *Iodine Deficiency Disorders in Livestock: Ecology and Economics*, Oxford University Press, England, 1997.

Pavelka, S., et al., "Bromide Kinetics and Distribution in the Rat. II Distribution of Bromide in the Body." *Biol Trace Res*, 2000.

Porter, P. Brynberg, *Transactions of the American Therapeutics Society*, F. A. Davis Co., Phila., 1910; Waring, E. J., MD, *Practical Therapeutics: Considered Chiefly with Reference to the Materia Medica*, Lindsay and Blakeston, PA, 1874.

Reid, H. A., *The Use of Iodine and Its Compounds in Veterinary Practice*, De Grucy and Co., LTD., London, circa 1936.

Reid, H. A., *The Uses of Iodine and its Compounds in Veterinary Medicine*, London, circa 1930.

Resin: Clinical Application, *The Original Internist*, 2006.

SEER thyroid cancer statistics and graphs courtesy of the NIH.

She, J., et al., "Polybrominated diphenyl ethers (PBDEs) and polychlorinated biphenyls (PCBs) in breast milk from the Pacific Northwest." *Chemosphere,* 67 (2007).

She, J., et al., "PBDEs in the San Francisco Bay Area: measurements in harbor seal blubber and human breast adipose tissue." *Chemosphere,* 2002, Feb; 46(5):697-707.

Shevin, W., Iodine Conference presentations, 2007.

Shishodia, S., "Guggulsterone inhibits tumor cell proliferation." *Biochemical Pharmacology,* Volume 74, Issue 1, 30 June, 2007.

Smyth, P. P., "Role of Iodine in Antioxidant Defense in Thyroid and Breast Disease." *Biofactors,* 2003; Coochi, M., et al., "A New Hypothesis of Bio-Chemical Cooperation?" *Prog Nutr,* 2000.

Stanbury J. B., (ed), *The Damaged Brain of Iodine Deficiency: Cognitive, Behavioral, Neuromotor, Educative Aspects,* Cognizant Communication Corporation, 1993.

Stiffler, L., "PBDes: They are everywhere, they accumulate and they spread." *Seattle Post-Intelligencer,* March 28, 2007.

Teas, J., et al., "Dietary Seaweed (Laminaria) and Mammary Carcinogens in Rats." *Cancer Res,* 1984.

Teas, J., et al., "Variability of Iodine Content in Common Commercially Available Edible Seaweeds." *Thyroid,* Volume 14, Number 10, 2004.

Tenpenny, S., Conversation at American Academy for the Advancement of Medicine Conference, 2005.

Tenpenny, S., YouTube video on Iodine at IAOMT Conference, 2007. *www.youtube.com/watch?v=hMjKmi12UX0.*

Thrall, K. D., "Differences in the Distribution of Iodine and Iodide in the Sprague-Dawley Rats." *J Toxicol Environ Health,* 1992.

Vega-Riveroll, L., et al., "Apoptotic and Antiproliferative Effects of Iodine Supplements on Human Breast Cancer Tumors." Poster, Thyroid Conference, New York, October, 2007.

Velicky, J., et al., "Long Term Action of Potassium Bromide on the Rat Thyroid Gland." *Acta Histochem,* 1998.

Velicky, J., et al., "Potassium Bromide and the Thyroid Gland of the Rat," *Morphology and Immunochemistry,* 1997.

Velicky, J., et al., "Potassium Bromide and the Thyroid Gland of the Rat," *Morphology and Immunochemistry,* RIA and INAA Analysis. *Ann Anat,* 1997, *www.credocluster.info,* Issue 6, July, 2006.

Velicky, J., et al., "The Effect of Bromide on the Ultrastructure of Rat Thyrocytes." *Ann Anat,* 2004.

Venturi, S., "Is There a Role for Iodine in Breast Disease?" *The Breast* 2001.

Vobecky, M., et al., "Interaction of Bromine with Iodine in the Rat Thyroid Gland at Enhanced Bromide Intake." *Biol Trace Elem Res*, 1996.

Web Internet References:
www.alibaba.com/catalog/11292709/sodium_bromate_99_5.html
www.gulflink.osd.mil/library/randrep/pb_paper/mr1018.2chap10.html
www.healthycar.org/chemicals.bromine.php
www.healthy-communications.com/hazards_of_cosmetics_by_carol_barzac95.html
www.healthytoys.org/chemicals.other.php

Where to Get Iodine

Where to find iodine supplements?

As the author, I highly recommend buying discount Iodoral and the iodine companion nutrients from our Breast Cancer Choices charity.

Please support this good cause at:

www.BreastCancerChoices.org/order

The fundraising shop is the main way we fund our Iodine Investigation Project for breast cancer patients, as well as providing other free educational materials.

Thank you for your support.

Index

breasts, 11, 34, 52, 52-6, 69-70, 74, 76, 85, 89-92, 95, 117, 128, 138, 168-9, 173, 177-8, 181-3, 189-90, 194, 214, 216
  iodine deficient, 89
bromate, 99,165-6, 177, 180, 209-12, 219, 223-5
  banned, 99, 210, 223
bromide, 25-6, 29, 31, 42, 53, 71, 81-2, 87, 89, 97-9, 100, 179-81, 196, 201, 203-5, 207-13, 216, 219-25
  iodine detoxing, 214
  trapped, 82
Bromide Dominance Theory, 207
bromide toxicity, salt water treatment for Gulf War soldiers, 73, 87
bromine/bromide-containing products competing with iodine, 217
bromine-saturated environment, 26, 195
bromism, misdiagnosed, 209
bromism symptoms, 25, 216
Brownstein, David, MD, 19, 21, 38, 43, 67, 72, 88, 93, 105, 142, 147, 153, 175, 201, 215-18, 224
  his book, *Iodine: Why You need It and Why You Can't Live Without It*, 216
  his book, *Salt Your Way to Health*, 88

C

calcifications, iodine supplementation helps resolve, 91-2, 161, 214
Canada, has banned bromate in bread, 99, 210, 223
cancer, 11-13, 15-21, 23, 25-6, 28, 38-9, 46, 50-1, 54, 56, 65-6, 68, 73-4, 77, 85, 89, 91, 93-5, 100, 128-30, 132, 136, 142, 154-7, 160-1, 170, 173-7,180-91, 200, 202, 205, 208-10, 213-18, 223-4
candida, 6, 55, 143, 146-7
cells
  all require iodine, 47, 49, 178, 215
  human breast cancer, and iodine-rich seaweed, 215
Celtic Sea Salt, recommended over refined salt, 34, 45, 190
chloride, competes with iodine, 167-8
Civil War and iodine use, 20, 117, 129, 138, 158
companion nutrients to iodine, 39, 45-6, 61, 63-5, 71-3, 88-9, 184, 201, 205
cosmetics and bromine/bromide additives, 211-12, 220-1, 224-5
Courtois, Bernard, French chemist, discoverer of iodine, 126, 136
Curezone, 94, 146
Curezone Iodine Forum, 23-4, 82, 93-4, 141, 154, 205
Curezoners, 23-4, 94
cysts, 6, 20, 22, 33, 50, 52, 69, 70, 74, 76, 78, 89, 128, 139, 170, 177-8, 181, 216

D

Dach, Jeffrey, MD, on selenium use with Hashimoto's Thyroiditis, 51
DeLong, G. Robert, MD, using iodine, savior of health of rural Chinese province (*see also* Xinjiang Province, China), 132
depression, a consistent complaint, among iodine stories, 33, 37, 42, 44, 53, 113, 144, 154, 204, 209, 216

Grass Roots Iodine Movement, 27,
32, 69, 94, 196

H

hair loss, 42, 46, 85, 161, 204
Hashimoto's disease and iodine, 51,
124, 170
headaches, 5, 7, 22, 45, 65, 81, 110,
113, 228
hemorrhoids and iodine
supplementation, 57, 61, 139
herpes, 37, 56, 114
Hippocrates, 15, 121, 136
history of iodine, 111, 117, 141,
157
hypothyroid, 75, 85, 90, 143-4, 151

I

information, medical, 16, 155
iodine
absorption of, 50, 66, 69, 71, 82
antidote for toxic bromine, 27,
182
as an antiseptic, 31, 35, 110, 130,
139, 149
body metabolizing, 74
bromine competes with, 167
bromine purges, 178
companion nutrients, 39, 45-6, 61,
63-5, 71-3, 88-9, 184, 201, 205
dangers of (see Wolff-Chaikoff
Effect)
decolorized, 50
desensitizes estrogen receptors,
183, 213, 215
discovered from seaweed ashes,
125-6
elemental, 50, 100, 114
given breast cancer patients after
biopsy, 183-4
Goiter Standards, 169
injected, 128, 139

molecular, and breast cancer, 218
nutritional vs. the antiseptic
form, 31
overpowered by bromine, 68
povidone, toxic, 49
purged by anti-iodine bromine,
25-6, 196
scorned as dangerous, 165
and secreting organs, 115
storing by thyroid and breast, 36
vapors treated lung ailments in
1820s, 137
white, 50
wrong, for women, 168
Iodine and Breast Cancer by Jonathan
Wright, MD, 157, 215
iodine and iodide, terms
interchangeable here, 29, 97,
224
iodine babies, 94
Iodine-based Medicine Time Line,
136
iodine canteen, used in Civil War,
128-9, 158
Iodine Conferences, 59, 63, 68, 142,
199, 201-203
iodine consumption
average, 164
sharply down in US, 25, 28, 167,
213-14
iodine content in seaweed, 38,
215
Iodine Crisis
current underlying cause, 196
epidemic, 31, 193
iodine deficiency, extreme, a cause,
178
iodine-deficiency conditions, 199
iodine-deficient state, and the
breast and thyroid, 190
iodine detox symptoms, 204
iodine detoxing, 71

Index

About the Author

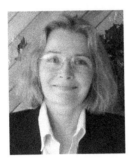

Lynne Farrow is a whistle blower. She is also a journalist, researcher, former college professor and speaker. Her own personal experience with breast cancer led to the discovery that someone had stolen a medicine with proven benefits reaching back 15,000 years. A medicine that not only helped her, but has helped millions.

She currently serves as Director of Breast Cancer Choices, Inc., a nonprofit organization dedicated to scrutinizing the evidence for breast cancer procedures and treatments.

As the founder of Breast Cancer Think Tank, she created a forum for professionals, patients and lay-people to report new findings about breast cancer as well as review old information with a friendly spirit of cooperation, challenge and debate.

Lynne is the editor of *www.IodineResearch.com*, where she has compiled materials for both beginning and advanced iodine investigators. From obscure studies on iodine and the brain, to information for the beginner looking for the widely accepted Iodine Protocol, the iodine research website provides a wealth of information.

www.LynneFarrow.net

Working with the Author

Lynne Farrow speaks to groups as small as ten or as large as 1,000 on the various topics listed in *The Iodine Crisis*. She also consults privately with individuals seeking scholarly resources or general background on iodine.

Visit *www.LynneFarrow.net* for more information.

Please Join the Discussion on the Iodine Workshop Facebook Group:

www.facebook.com/groups/IodineWorkshop

9 780986 032004